Endorsements

"Of the numerous publications on the pros and cons of immunization, Dr. Davis presents a refreshing side. At last an alternative to immunization! A must-read book for those who are deliberating on what to do if you do not want to opt for immunization—and even for those who have had immunization. A timely, recommended book that every traveler, health worker, missionary, and health-conscious citizen should have information about."—Ruth Mariano, M.D. (Philippines)

"Preventive medicine involves building the body's defenses against possible attack by pathogens. In that sense, inoculation (vaccination) can be more causitive than preventive, as it introduces the pathogen into the system. This book shows that true prevention will thus utilize diet and positive health habits to reinforce the immune system."—Dorcas Ayayo, M.D. (Kenya)

"After having read several books (and this one) on the very controversial issue of vaccination and immunity, I believe that we maybe, probably, possibly—not being fully given the transparent facts of this potential help or hazard by the powers that be—should make utmost effort to keep our immune systems always operating at par. I think every serious and conscientious parent should have *Vaccine Alternatives* foremost in their health library."—Cherie Lou N. Fernandez, M.D., FPOGS (Philippines)

"This book makes clear that an emotional, personal great debate is going on regarding the use of vaccines. Many answers are offered to a lot of questions about vaccine use and their potential risk. The clear options show how important it is to strengthen the body's natural immunity to common diseases with healthy lifestyle practices."—Yohannas Gamlak, M.D. (Ethiopia)

VACCINE

ALTERNATIVES

How to Prevent and Treat Illness
Using Natural Remedies

An Essential Guide for Patients, Parents,
Travelers, and Healthcare Workers

Ervin Davis, M.D.

PRINTED IN U.S.A.
Hagerstown, Maryland

ISBN 978-0-615-19347-2

Obtain additional copies of this book by contacting
Ervin Davis, M.D.
P. O. Box 6276
Thomasville, GA 31758
E-mail: ervhealthylifestyle@gmail.com

About the Author

Ervin Davis was born in South Georgia. He grew up on a farm with loving parents and an extended family. After serving in the U.S. Army during the Vietnam era, he attended Atlantic Union College, majoring in biology and religion. He studied medicine at the University of Montemorelos School of Medicine and Universidad De Americana Del Norte in Mexico.

Dr. Davis has been a medical researcher at the University of Massachusetts Medical Center and the Long Island Jewish Medical Center in the departments of surgery, pediatric urology, and pharmacology/anesthesiology. He was an adjunct professor and director of the Pre-Professional Advisory Program at Florida A&M University and a founding faculty member of the Florida State University College of Medicine. He enjoys teaching students to become medical missionary practitioners.

He is also executive director of Healthy Lifestyle Choices Inc., a Georgia-based non-profit organization established in 1993 to promote better health, with primary emphasis on health education, disease prevention, and lifestyle improvement. This organization educates primarily rural communities in the prevention of lifestyle-induced diseases, such as heart attack, hypertension, stroke, diabetes, cirrhosis of the liver, formation of gallstones, obesity, and other illnesses. In addition, the organization addresses such topics as stress management, nutrition education, and the dangers of smoking, drinking, and overeating. An area of special concern is the childhood obesity epidemic.

Ervin and his wife, Lynn, are teachers at heart and partners in ministry. Lynn teaches middle school students and assists with conducting Weekend Wellness Seminars.

Author's Note

The author assumes responsibility for all facts and opinions cited in this book.

The health and medical information in this book is not intended for use as specific treatment for a specific condition. Symptoms and diseases vary with individuals and should be evaluated by your healthcare provider.

The purpose of this book is to help readers prevent disease, enact lifestyle changes, and improve their general well-being.

Thanks

With gratitude I acknowledge all who participated in the creation of this book. The many hours spent researching, proofreading, editing, and designing are greatly appreciated. Thank you.

Table of Contents

Why Should You Care About Vaccines?

To vaccinate or not to vaccinate? The question terrifies both parents and patients. By refusing a vaccination, do I risk exposing my infant to a deadly or disabling illness? By accepting the injection, do I accept a different risk—that of introducing toxins and foreign genetic material into the body of a developing child? So much hysteria surrounds the vaccination issue that both options seem risky.

Most parents and patients react by giving up; they take the shots, but worry secretly whether they did the right thing. Or they opt out of the vaccination plan, but constantly fret about what to do if their family members do contract a contagious illness. Just the thought that you are giving a lifelong legacy to your child is a fearful one.

The vaccination issue causes controversy not only in North America but around the world. Deciding whether or not to receive vaccinations is a serious and, ultimately, a personal matter. Only you can make an informed, thoughtful decision for yourself and your family. Moreover, when international travelers and missionaries prepare to embark, they face a "roll of the dice." Just think, when the trip is over, it may not truly be over because of long-term complications from a tropical disease.

We now understand that all vaccines can potentially cause a reaction in some children and adults. For many, the frightening side effects are worse than the disease itself. Even many of the common vaccines have been associated with serious side effects, including neurological complications, seizures, dermatitis, fever, encephalitis, retinopathy, blindness, joint pain, and death.

Further, opponents of immunization remind us that the long-term effects of vaccinations are not known. Some propose that there may be a real correlation between early immunization and the later development of mental problems, learning disabilities, autism, hyperactivity, and depression of the immune system.

In addition to citing potential health effects, opponents question the efficacy of vaccines in the first place. As an example, some observe that measles outbreaks have been known to course through school populations despite the fact that nearly 100 percent of the students had been immunized against the disease. Studies have shown that up to 10 percent of children who were vaccinated against pertussis (whooping cough) go on to contract the disease anyway.

The conclusion of conscientious patients and caregivers around the world is clear: immunity is more than immunization.

What can we do? We can boost resistance to disease by supporting and enhancing the natural immune system; first, by breastfeeding infants (a mother's immunities are temporarily transferred to her baby this way), and later, by providing a nutritious diet and immune-enhancing supplements. We can create stress-free, loving, and nurturing home environments. We can avoid high-risk environments such as daycare, large elementary schools, and crowded shopping mall settings. Finally, we can return to the healing power of medicinal plants. These have been used to prevent and treat disease for centuries and still play an important role in cultures around the planet. With such simple and reasonable options, we can actively promote health and well-being.

I am not the only voice in the chorus of concern about conventional vaccinations. In the past decade, news programs, magazine features, websites, and an increasing number of books have sounded a warning call about the risks of injecting bacteria, viruses, toxins, chemicals, and drugs into the body or bloodstream. So what makes this book different? Instead of just pointing out what's wrong with common immunization programs, I want to point you toward something right. I'll explain how current scientific research supports specific natural remedies that will improve your immunity to disease and help you fight common illnesses if you do contract them. Do you want to learn more? Keep reading.

Part I

Overview of Vaccination

Chapter 1

Questioning Vaccines? You're Not Alone

Many loving parents, travelers, and missionaries are saying no to medical vaccinations. Worldwide, concerned parents and caretakers of over 5 millions infants and children are making this decision each year. (Between 1995 and 2001, more than 2.1 million American children between 19 and 35 months of age were not vaccinated or under-vaccinated. That number has steadily increased since the 2001 study.[1]) After considerable personal research, some families have chosen to change whether or how they receive vaccinations. However, many in the medical profession and the government say that such a decision is dangerous and based upon erroneous conclusions, ignorance, poverty, or conspiracy paranoia; some even suggest it constitutes a form of child abuse. Some have attempted to usurp the fundamental rights of citizens by mandating vaccination.

Today, the decision not to vaccinate is no longer odd and has developed into a worldwide anti-vaccination movement. Conscientious healthcare professionals, scientists, and the unvaccinated population have taken the lead at an ever-increasing rate. Magazines and books are filled with material on the subject. Courageous health providers put their professional lives on the line by daring to question and go against conventional immunization practices.

This book is not intended to sway your opinion one way or another about conventional vaccinations. It will, however, help clarify why natural alternatives may be preferable to conventional vaccinations. The author is mainly concerned with safety and hopes to provide an alternative approach with natural remedies that are effective and appropriate. In the case of vaccinations, the serious question is whether the benefits really outweigh the risks.

As you will see, we have many natural options for protecting against infectious disease with nutrition, vitamins, herbs, and a healthy lifestyle. Recently, much attention has been placed on supportive scientific research and documentation for these alternatives, and readers are encouraged to look into the many references provided so as to more fully understand the debate and available options.

A growing body of anecdotal and scientific evidence indicates that vaccines may not be as safe or as effective as previously claimed. In fact, a growing number of studies have pointed to the conclusion that vaccines sometimes represent a dangerous assault on the immune system, possibly leading to autoimmune diseases such as multiple sclerosis, lupus, juvenile onset diabetes, dermatitis, fibromyalgia, and chronic fatigue syndrome, as well as previously rare disorders such as brain cancer, childhood leukemia, sudden infant death syndrome (SIDS), autism, and asthma. It is neither ethical nor wise to sacrifice a single child when such doubts exist regarding the current vaccine system.

As you read these pages and make your decision about vaccinations, you are strongly encouraged to read what various experts have to say and draw your own conclusions. Do not rely solely on the advice of your doctors, but do ask your doctor and other healthcare professionals about the risks and possible side effects, then complement this information with what you read.

Vaccine Dogma Challenged

Many in the medical community regard vaccinations as an unquestioned dogma, never to be challenged or refused for any reason. Like antibiotics, cancer chemotherapy, the annual physical, mammograms, and Pap tests, the validity of vaccinations and their effectiveness require a second look. Vaccination is a medical treatment, and, like dogmas, assumptions regarding the effectiveness of medical practices abound. However, we are obligated to pay attention when parents make thousands of statements like this one: *"My child was normal, happy, and healthy. He was walking, learning to talk, and interacting with his siblings. He was normal in every way until his one-year well-baby check up. The doctor said it was time for his next round of shots. Without questions, the shots were given. Within weeks, he was autistic."*

The reports and observations vary slightly in content and timing, but the descriptions of thousands of children who suddenly regress into the isolated world of autism are eerily the same. Conscientious members of the medical community and society are reinvestigating scientific claims passed on as dogma and are seeing some of these claims crumble when challenged by scientific fact.

Although autism has been cited by public health officials and autism researchers to occur in 2 to 10 out of 10,000 children nationwide, the Centers for Disease Control released a report in April 2000 showing the incidence of autism in Brick Township, New Jersey, in 1998 to be 1 in 150 children. Likewise, the incidence in the Granite Bay, California, public elementary school district is 1 in 132 children. These statistics may be more reflective of the true rate of autism in the U.S. today. The Autism Society of America estimates that "more than one-half million people in the U.S. today have autism or some form of pervasive developmental disorder," making autism one of the most common developmental disabilities.[2]

Parental fears about vaccine risks are not alleviated when the U.S. Government's Vaccine Injury Compensation program has paid over half a billion dollars since its inception for vaccine-related injuries and death. In addition to this fear, consider that fewer than 10 percent of doctors even report vaccine-related problems.

Vaccines carry the risk of injury or death and yet are practically forced upon every healthy citizen. Until the late 1980s, few questioned the wisdom of this lucrative pharmaceutical enterprise. Regardless of the scare tactics and rhetoric, the fact is that parents in the United States and some other parts of the world have the legal right to refuse vaccinations for themselves and their children.

All states in the U.S. allow exemptions to compulsory vaccinations for medical reasons, and most allow exemptions for religious or philosophical/personal beliefs. Anyone telling you otherwise is uninformed or perhaps attempting to promote particular beliefs. (See Appendix for information on exemptions in the U.S.)

In recent years, the Centers for Disease Control (CDC), Federal Drug Administration (FDA), and other U.S. government agencies have been accused of supporting biased and questionable studies that were financed by vaccine manufacturers and promoting compulsory medical vaccination of healthy children and adults. There is also the matter of conflict of interest existing among employees with a vested interest in research results. According to some who have analyzed the studies, many pro-vaccination papers are statistically flawed and illogical. Further, studies designed to look at the long-term effect of vaccines are virtually nonexistent. Millions of dollars and much political power are wrapped up in the advancement of the vaccination debate, so it is increasingly unlikely that the negative aspects of vaccines will be admitted. It is up to individuals to probe for the truth.

Vaccines Work Against the Body's Natural Processes

Natural-remedies practitioners believe vaccines work against natural processes and thwart the body's natural ability to fight off disease. By suppressing our immunity, vaccines actually make more diseases available to the body. Many normal diseases (such as measles, mumps, and chickenpox) enter the body by first making contact with nasal or oral

7

mucosa. White blood cells are activated to move and respond to those invading pathogens. The white blood cells increase movement in response to *chemotaxis* (a movement or orientation of cells along a chemical concentration gradient either toward or away from the chemical stimulus) and will leave the blood vessels to enter the area where they are needed. Many believe that childhood illnesses are important to the maturation and development of the immune system.

There is a school of thought that measles, mumps, rubella (German measles), and chickenpox, which enter the body through the mucous membranes, serve a necessary and positive purpose in challenging and strengthening the immune system of these membranes. In contrast, the respective vaccines of these diseases are injected by needle directly into the system of the child, thereby bypassing the mucosal immune system. As a result, mucosal immunity remains relatively weak and stunted in many children, a complication which may be linked to susceptibility to repeated upper respiratory infections and to the rapid increase in asthma and eczema now being seen.

Common childhood illnesses are believed by some to protect against more serious, life-threatening conditions. This theory suggests that if infections such as measles or chickenpox occur when antibodies against these viruses are already present (such as within the first few months after birth in the child who has been immunized), the immune system cannot react fully to the infection. This gives the virus the chance to become persistent and to develop later as an autoimmune disease or other chronic allergy problem.

Significantly, vaccinations may temporarily lower immune function. This observation is based on research which found that T-cell (white blood cell) ratios fell to low levels for up to two weeks after tetanus booster doses in apparently healthy persons.

Further, it is a common observation made by parents, pediatricians, and other clinical practitioners that children suffer more infections, colds, ear infections, and rhinitis just after vaccinations than do unvaccinated children. Unvaccinated children stand a much better chance at avoiding disease because no aspect of their immune system has been suppressed.

Can Vaccinations Cause Disease?

It is not the focus of this book to detail the many examples of ineffectiveness in vaccines, the negative reactions after injections, or the deaths as a result of immunizations. However, the following are some examples of immunization incidents, which will give you an idea of the scope of problems:

- In the 1970s a tuberculosis vaccine trial in India involving 260,000 people revealed that more cases of TB occurred in the vaccinated group than in the unvaccinated.[3]
- In the U.S., from July 1990 to November 1993, the U.S. Food and Drug Administration counted a total of 54,072 adverse reactions following vaccination. The FDA admitted that this number represented only about 10 percent of the real total because most doctors were not reporting vaccine injuries. In other words, adverse reactions for this period may have exceeded an incredible half a million.[4]
- It is a matter of public record that Jonas Salk, inventor of the injected polio vaccine, testified to a Senate subcommittee that the oral polio vaccine has caused most of the polio outbreaks since 1961.[5]
- The Ohio Department of Health reported that 2,720 children developed measles in 1989, despite the fact that close to three-quarters of the cases occurred in previously vaccinated children. The U.S. Centers for Disease Control and Prevention (CDC) even reported measles outbreaks in a documented 100-percent-vaccinated population. According to the CDC, among school-aged children, measles outbreaks have occurred in schools with vaccination levels greater than 98 percent. These outbreaks have occurred in all parts of the country, including areas that had not reported measles for years. In addition, half of the reported pertussis cases in Ohio from 1987 to 1991 occurred in children who were vaccinated.
- In 1979, Sweden abandoned the whooping cough vaccine due to its ineffectiveness. Out of 5,140 cases in 1978, it was found that 84 percent had been vaccinated three times.[6]

Are Vaccinations Necessary?

In many parts of the world, it has been observed that disease and death rates had already fallen dramatically prior to widespread vaccination. As an example, mortality from diphtheria was already reduced to fewer than 7 per 100,000 children by the mid-1940s, before the introduction of the vaccine. In addition, the morbidity and mortality rate for measles was already less than one per 100,000 infected in the mid-1950s, almost a decade before the vaccine was produced. Clearly, in both situations the diseases had already become less deadly before the introduction of vaccines.

Many experts observe that the declining occurrence of childhood diseases seems to parallel improved hygienic practices, sanitation, and improved water quality rather than vaccination programs. Prior to vaccinations in both the U.S. and westernized European countries, infectious disease death rates declined 85 percent and measles mortality declined

97 percent. Poverty, poor nutrition, crowded and unsanitary conditions, and a lack of access to medical care are far more likely to contribute to the development and spread of disease than the absence of a vaccine. Vaccine advocates admit that shots are not 100 percent effective. It has been observed that measles epidemics can occur in populations with an immunization rate close to 100 percent. Over the past 20 years, notable incidences have occurred in Warren County, Pennsylvania, and Juneau, Alaska, U.S.A.; in Fife, Scotland; in Geneva, Switzerland; and in Japan. This is despite a vaccination density of over 96 percent. Outbreaks of measles continue to occur in many parts of the world, even though there has been a high density of MMR vaccination.

Medical literature documents a surprisingly high incidence of vaccine failures for measles, mumps, polio, smallpox, influenza, and numerous other contagious diseases in vaccinated populations. One of the theories as to why this occurs is that vaccination results in immune suppression, which then creates an increased susceptibility to infections.

Types of Adverse Reactions

There are several general types of adverse effects, injuries, and complications that are associated with vaccinations. Some occur almost immediately after a child receives the injection; others may take hours, days, even months, or possibly years to appear.

Toxic

In vaccines that contain killed bacteria, the bacteria can release toxins into the bloodstream. If these toxins reach the brain, neurological problems, including autism, Attention Deficit Disorder (ADD), behavioral problems, and other syndromes could develop.

Autoimmune

Vaccines are supposed to trigger the body's immune system to attack the vaccine's components. Suppose the immune system attacks more than it is supposed to, say, a part of the body that is chemically similar to the vaccine? This type of reaction is called *autoimmune*, meaning that the body attacks itself. Such reactions have been reported for measles, tetanus, and flu vaccines.

Infectious

Vaccines that contain live viruses may actually cause the disease they are supposed to prevent. The oral polio vaccine was responsible for approximately 10 reported cases of polio each year it was given. As of January 1, 2000, the oral polio vaccine is no longer recommended. Also measles, mumps, rubella, and chickenpox vaccines sometimes lead to symptoms of diseases they were designed to prevent.

Vaccines: Recipe for Success or Tragedy?

One safety issue that is often overlooked when it comes to vaccines is the "recipe." All vaccines have three main types of ingredients:

- the "germ" material: killed or live viruses or bacteria, toxoids, or DNA
- ingredients that are added to perform a variety of functions
- the culture in which the vaccines are prepared

Let's look at these factors.

Wanted: Dead or Alive?

Vaccines have traditionally come in two basic forms: dead (inactivated or killed) or live (attenuated). The vast majority of both forms are delivered one of two ways: via injection under the skin (subcutaneous) or into the muscle (intramuscular). (Polio and typhoid vaccines are also available in oral form.) In some cases, both live and killed vaccines are available to treat the same disease. A third type of vaccine, the recombinant DNA vaccine, is the product of genetic engineering. It is the newest form, but questions remain about its safety and efficacy.

Live Vaccines

Live vaccines are made in a laboratory from the living organism (usually a virus) that causes the disease. Live vaccines are *attenuated*, or weakened, so they will cause the body's immune system to generate an immune response without (hopefully) causing the disease. Some people, however, do respond to a vaccination by developing symptoms of the disease, although in most cases they are mild. Examples of live attenuated virus vaccines include polio (oral), measles, mumps, chickenpox, rubella, and yellow fever. Live bacterial vaccines include one for typhoid fever and the Bacillus-Calmette-Guerin (BCG) vaccine, which is used for tuberculosis.

Some experts claim that the immune system responds to live attenuated vaccines the same way it does to a natural infection; others disagree. In fact, even proponents of live vaccines agree that live vaccines can cause a mild version of the disease they are designed to prevent. People who question the wisdom of giving live vaccines, especially to infants and young children, say these vaccines may have much more serious

11

consequences, pointing to a reported correlation with autism and auto-immune diseases.

Killed Vaccines

A killed, or inactivated, vaccine consists of all or part of the disease-causing organism, which has been killed or rendered inactive. Unlike live vaccines, killed vaccines cannot reproduce, so they are not able to cause the disease they are designed to prevent. They trigger a weaker response by the immune system than do live vaccines. They also tend to be safer than live vaccines for people who have a weakened immune system, for pregnant women, and for young children. Most killed vaccines are protein-based, like the bacteria they mimic. Some of these bacteria are coated with sugars called polysaccharides.

Recombinant DNA Vaccines

Another type of vaccine is a recombinant DNA (genetically engineered) vaccine. The hepatitis B vaccine is one example. Rather than using the entire organism, recombinant DNA vaccines are made by taking specific genes from the infectious agent (for example, virus or bacteria) and adding them to the vaccine culture. For example, hepatitis B vaccine is made by inserting a portion of the hepatitis B virus gene into baker's yeast, the culture in which this vaccine is produced.

Experts say recombinant DNA vaccines are more effective and safer than other types of vaccines because they don't contain the entire infectious agent and thus cannot cause an actual infection. However, the greatest concern about recombinant DNA vaccines is that they may cause the immune system to produce antibodies, which in turn attack parts of the body and cause health problems. Much is still not known about the effects of recombinant DNA vaccines.

Added Ingredients

Because of the immaturity of the child's immune system, parents need to look at the ingredients in vaccines and the dangers they may cause.

The "recipe" for the vaccines your child is taking may include the following ingredients:

Aluminum gels: This metal is added to vaccines, in the form of gels or salts, to promote the production of antibodies. Aluminum has been named as a possible cause of seizures, Alzheimer's disease, brain damage, dementia, and other nervous system disorders. These substances have also been associated with reactions like erythema and subcutaneous nodules. Aluminum is used in the DTaP and hepatitis B vaccines.

Benzethonium chloride: The anthrax vaccine (given primarily to military personnel) contains this ingredient. It is a preservative and has not been evaluated for human consumption.

Ethylene glycol: This is the main ingredient in antifreeze. It is used in some vaccines (for example, DTaP, polio, Hib, and hepatitis B) as a preservative.

Formaldehyde: This substance is of great concern because it is a known carcinogen (cancer-causing agent). Formaldehyde is perhaps best known for its use in the embalming process, but it is also used in fungicides, insecticides, and in the manufacture of explosives and fabrics. In vaccines, liquid formaldehyde, called formalin, is used to inactivate germs. Formaldehyde may be found in several vaccines.

Gelatin: This known allergen is found in the varicella and MMR vaccines. It is often made from the muscle fiber of animals.

Glutamate: This substance, a known nervous excitotoxin, is used to stabilize some vaccines against heat, light, and other environmental conditions. It is known to cause adverse reactions such as nausea, dizziness, headaches, and diarrhea, and is found in the varicella vaccine.

Neomycin: This antibiotic is used to prevent germs from growing in the vaccine cultures. Neomycin can cause allergic reactions in some people. It is found in the MMR and the polio (IPV) vaccines.

Streptomycin: This antibiotic is known to cause allergic reactions in some people. It is found in both forms of the polio vaccine.

Sulfites: Sodium metabisulfite is a preservative also found in many foods and some alcoholic beverages. Large oral doses of sulfites can cause shortness of breath, wheezing, diarrhea, vomiting, cramps, and dizziness.

Phenol: This coal-tar derivative is used in the production of dyes, disinfectants, plastics, preservatives, and germicides. It is highly poisonous in certain doses and actually harms rather than stimulates the immune system, which is the exact opposite of what vaccines are designed to do. Phenol is used in the preparation of some vaccines, including typhoid.

Thimerosal: This substance, a known allergen and poison, is a preservative that contains nearly 50 percent ethyl mercury, which means it has many of the same properties mercury has; thus, it is very toxic. For decades it was used in nearly every vaccine on the market. Most childhood vaccines in the U.S. are now offered in single doses, which are thimerosal-free except for trace amounts. Manufacturers are working to remove those traces. As of February 2008, none of the recommended childhood vaccines, except influenza, will contain thimerosal. The American Academy of Pediatrics (AAP) and the U.S. Public Health Service (PHS) released a joint statement acknowledging the dangers of thimerosal.

Although the above ingredients are present in minuscule amounts in vaccines, they are, for the most part, poisons or known allergens (for which no safe amount has been established). Once they are injected into your child's bloodstream and immature immune system, they are not adequately eliminated by the bile and the liver because bile production has not yet matured.

Vaccine Cultures

Patients rarely stop to think about the fact that vaccines introduce foreign genetic material to the body. For vaccines that are not genetically engineered (as are the hepatitis B vaccine and many of the vaccines now under development), a toxic bacterium or a live virus is weakened by repeatedly passing it through a culture medium, such as human cells (aborted fetus tissue), monkey kidney tissue, chicken/duck embryo, guinea pig embryo cells, or calf serum, in order to reduce the organism's potency.

Killed vaccines are inactivated using chemicals, heat, or radiation. The weakened virus or bacterium is then strengthened by adding stabilizers and adjuvants, which are substances that boost the antibody production in the vaccine (such as those named under "Added Ingredients").

Potential dangers may be introduced during the making of most vaccines. All viruses, dead and alive, contain DNA and RNA, the carriers of genetic material. When vaccines are made, these viruses are placed in a culture medium, which may include rabbit brain tissue, guinea pig tissue, dog kidney tissue, monkey kidney tissue, chicken embryo, or chicken or duck egg protein. The RNA and DNA from the viruses can be picked up by the animal cells in the culture. Cells in which the viral RNA integrates into the DNA of the animal cells are called pro-viruses.

Pro-viruses may lie dormant (inactive) in the body for long periods of time. If they become active, many expert bacteriologists and virologists believe they are responsible for autoimmune disorders, in which the immune system cannot distinguish between its own tissues and foreign invaders. Hence, the body attacks itself. Examples of autoimmune diseases include asthma, rheumatoid arthritis, diabetes, multiple sclerosis, and systemic lupus erythematosus (SLE). In addition, the animal proteins (tissue is composed of proteins) used in the cultures are not digested in the human body, and undigested proteins are a major cause of allergies. Undigested proteins can also attack the protective covering on the nerve cells and cause neurological problems, such as multiple sclerosis.

Moreover, another kind of tissue in which some vaccines are grown is human fetal tissue. At least one each of the polio, MMR, rabies, chickenpox, and hepatitis A vaccines are made in this manner. The important question of whether these vaccines can cause an autoimmune response once they are injected has not been definitively answered and deserves further study. The use of human fetal tissue is also an ethical issue for many people.

Vaccines and Autoimmune Diseases?

The medical community, governmental agencies, and the pharmaceutical complex push widespread immunization despite incomplete knowledge of what vaccines do to the immune system. As an example, it has been frequently observed that antibody levels do not correspond with immunity to the disease for which the vaccination was given. The potential disease-provoking properties of a vaccine are largely unknown, and autoimmune disease may be the end result of damage caused by vaccines.

A causal connection between vaccinations and the onset of autoimmune disease remains to be proven. However, a growing number of researchers and clinicians have argued that conditions such as juvenile rheumatoid arthritis could be the body's reaction to foreign pathogens or protein contained in vaccines. As stated above, the body's immune system is designed to defend against infectious disease-causing organisms. When presented with a foreign pathogen or protein, the immune system mobilizes to fight off the "enemy."

Over time the immune system comes to "memorize" a number of invaders and can, therefore, respond quickly to an intruder. However, certain foreign substances—vaccines, for example—may have a similar structure as some body tissue; as a result, the antibodies that are produced to attack the pathogens in the vaccine could also lead to the immune system attacking body tissue with a similar structure. It is this lack of differentiation between the body's own tissue and foreign cells that leads to autoimmune diseases.

The Immature Immune System

Infants come into the world with antibodies they have received from their mothers through the placenta. Infants who are breastfed continue to receive many important antibodies in the colostrum (the thick, yellowish pre-milk that is secreted during the first seven days after a woman gives birth) and breast milk.

The problem many doctors and parents have with vaccines is that an infant's or child's immune system cannot adequately respond to a vaccine. Many experts believe it takes at least six months for this to begin to happen.

Vaccines and Childhood Allergies?

Asthma, chronic fatigue syndrome, eczema, fibromyalgia, hay fever, multiple sclerosis, and psoriasis have all been associated with chemical and food allergies. Many pediatricians blame the rising incidence of these allergic conditions on the early ingestion of allergenic foods. The early introduction of allergens has been documented to increase the incidence of chronic allergic illness.

Despite these observations, children at a very early age are systematically exposed to foreign proteins (allergens) in the form of immunizations. It is a contradiction for doctors on one hand to advise parents to avoid early childhood contact with allergens and, on the other hand, to promote vaccinations that expose children to allergens and foreign protein.

With the growing severity and debilitation of immune diseases in children, especially asthma, should we not first conduct studies to determine the connection between immunizations and subsequent immune system impairment and destruction? Conventional medical authorities demand proof of the safety and efficacy of natural remedies before they are recommended for children. Why isn't the same proof demanded for vaccinations?

Admittedly, other factors in highly industrialized societies may be influencing the increase of autoimmune disorders (environmental factors, pesticides in food and water, use of animal products, and so on). We would do well to remain vigilant and pursue all possible culprits that could endanger our families and children.

Chapter 2

What is an Acceptable Risk?

S o now we've examined the recent attacks on vaccines, including the concern that their widespread and frequent use can lead to adverse reactions and long-term health disorders. But what about the other side? Some conclude that the risks of certain diseases far outweigh the risks associated with the vaccination process. Unfortunately, for those who comprise the high-risk group for serious vaccine reactions, the advantages offered by vaccines are understandably overshadowed by fears of debilitating or even fatal adverse reactions.

As you read this chapter, you are challenged to consider the risks of disease versus the risks of shots. It is important that you weigh this risk-to-benefit ratio carefully for yourself and your family.

Childhood Immunization Schedule (BABY SHOTS)
What follows is a description of each shot in the routine childhood immunization schedule. This list includes the age recommendations and risk factors connected with each vaccine.

POLIO Vaccine:
1.   First dose at 2 months
2.   Second dose at 4 months
3.   Third dose at 6 to 18 months
4.   Fourth dose at 4 to 6 years

POLIO: What is the risk for a child developing paralytic disease and meningitis associated with poliomyelitis? Even under epidemic conditions, natural polio produces no symptoms in over 90 percent of those exposed to it.[7] There have been no cases of wild polio in the U.S. in the past 20 years. Those cases which have been documented have been caused by the vaccine.[8]

The following side effects of the vaccine are possible:

With killed virus polio: Reactions can include fever of 102° F. in up to 38 percent, sleepiness, fussiness, crying, decreased appetite, vomiting, Guillain-Barré Syndrome, and allergic reaction in those allergic to neomycin, polymyxin B, and streptomycin. Precautions include those who have had a previous negative reaction, pregnant women, and possibly those with HIV/AIDS or otherwise compromised immune systems. **With live virus polio:** Reactions can include contraction of polio by those who have received the virus and by those who come into contact with body fluids and wastes of the immunized person. Paralytic symptoms may follow contraction of polio. Live virus is reportedly shed for up to eight weeks after the inoculation. Guillain-Barré Syndrome has also been noted. Not recommended for use in households where someone has a compromised immune system, for pregnant women, or where a previous reaction has been reported.[9]

Killed virus Ipol is grown on monkey kidney cells and contains formaldehyde and triple antibiotics. Poliovax is grown on cells from an aborted fetus and contains formaldehyde, cow serum, and triple antibiotic solution.[10] The monkey kidney cells used in the original killed polio vaccine contain SV40 (a virus that causes cancers in monkeys and that is used widely in genetic and medical research) and have been found in tumor cells of children whose parents were vaccinated against polio using the contaminated virus.[11] The live vaccine is grown on monkey kidney cells, antibiotics, and calf serum.

HAEMOPHILUS INFLUENZAE B (Hib) Vaccine:
1. First dose at 2 months
2. Second dose at 4 months
3. Third dose at 6 months
4. Fourth dose at 12 to 15 months

HAEMOPHILUS INFLUENZAE B: What is the risk of a child developing meningitis (although this vaccine will not protect the child from meningitis from all other forms such as pneumococcus, meningococcus, viruses, and fungi), pneumonia, and infections of the blood, joints, bone, and soft tissue associated with Haemophilus Influenzae B? This disease is most likely to occur in children up to 15 months of age and is fatal in 3 to 6 percent of children who contract it. Incidence of this disease today is low, and the vaccine has not proven to be highly effective in 41 percent of cases, according to some studies.[12] Treatment is available. The vaccine is often combined with the DTaP, which has the highest reaction rate of any vaccine available today. Adverse reactions can include contracting Hib, localized pain, erythema and induration, fever greater than 100.6, irritability, lethargy, anorexia, rhinorrhea, diarrhea, vomiting, and cough, when administered alone. Reactions occurred in up to 30 percent of patients. When administered in conjunction with the DTaP, reactions include local tenderness, erythema and induration, fever greater than

100.8, irritability, drowsiness, anorexia, diarrhea, vomiting, persistent crying, seizures, urticaria, hives, renal failure, Guillain-Barré Syndrome, and death. Reactions occurred in up to 77.9 percent of patients.[13]

The vaccine contains yeast, thimerosal (mercury derivative), and diphtheria toxoid when given alone.[14]

DIPHTHERIA, PERTUSSIS AND TETANUS (DTaP) Vaccine:
1. First dose at 2 months
2. Second dose at 4 months
3. Third dose at 6 months
4. Fourth dose at 15 to 18 months
5. Fifth dose at 4 to 6 years old
6. Booster doses at 11 or 12 years of age and older

PERTUSSIS: What is the risk of a child developing whooping cough, pneumonia, convulsions, inflammation of the brain, and death associated with pertussis? The disease is rarely fatal, with a 99.8 percent recovery rate. It is most serious and life-threatening in children under six months old, but there are adequate methods of treatment available.[15] The vaccine is most often given in conjunction with diphtheria and tetanus as the DTaP, which replaces the old DPT vaccine. The older DPT caused especially serious side effects; one patient in 600 suffered a severe reaction in one study,[16] and one in 875 suffered shock-collapse and convulsions.[17] Those in the second study were only tracked for the first 48 hours following immunization. Another study indicated that one in 100 reacted with convulsions, collapse, or high-pitched screaming, and one in three of those cases sustained permanent brain damage.[18] In a study of 103 children who died of SIDS, 70 percent died within three weeks of the DPT vaccine, and 37 percent of those died within the first week.[19]

The modified DTaP vaccine was released in 1996. In some cases it may be abbreviated DaPT. This version is called "acellular" pertussis (or aP) and is considered purer than the older, whole-cell pertussis vaccine. The "old" pertussis vaccine still contained a killed form of the whole pertussis bacteria. Manufacturers now take advantage of recent advances in protein chemistry and protein purification techniques. The DTaP is recommended as a safer option for vaccination, though it is not without problems. Side effects of this shot were only tracked for 72 hours and included tenderness, erythema, induration, fever greater than 102.2, drowsiness, fretfulness, vomiting, upper respiratory infection, diarrhea, rash, febrile seizures, persistent or unusual crying (hypotonic-hyporesponsive episode), lethargy, urticaria, anaphylactic shock, convulsions, encephalopathy, mono- and polyneuropathies, and death.[20] *DTaP vaccines contain trace amounts of formaldehyde and aluminum phosphate, and outside the U.S. they may contain thimerosal (mercury derivative).* [21]

DIPHTHERIA: What is the risk of a child developing paralysis, heart failure, or respiratory failure associated with diphtheria? To date only five cases have been reported annually since 1980.[22] Diphtheria is rarely fatal and can be treated with natural remedies or antibiotics and bed rest.[23] The diphtheria component is most often given within the DTaP and includes the same side effects and reactions as those listed for pertussis.

TETANUS: What is the risk for a child of developing fatal neuromuscular disease related to tetanus? It is understood that the incidence of tetanus is low, and there is an antitoxin that can be given in emergency situations, should we decline the immunization. Contracting tetanus does not provide lifelong immunity and neither does the vaccine. I understand that to prevent more severe reactions from the vaccine, the tetanus component has been so significantly "diluted" that it is clinically ineffective.[24] The death rate for properly treated cases of tetanus may be as high as 20 percent.[25] Side effects of the tetanus vaccine alone include high fever, pain, recurrent abscess formation, inner ear nerve damage, demyelinating neuropathy, anaphylactic shock, and loss of consciousness.[26] Tetanus given in the DPT or DTaP shot includes the same side effects and reactions as those listed for pertussis.

A new vaccine, called Tdap, is different from the DTaP vaccine currently given to babies and young children. It is given to adolescents and adults as a booster shot. Tdap contains fewer quantities of diphtheria and pertussis proteins; for this reason, Tdap is much less likely than DTaP to cause side effects such as pain, redness, and tenderness in adolescents.

MEASLES (RUBEOLA), MUMPS, RUBELLA (MMR) Vaccine:
1. First dose at 12 to 15 months
2. Second dose at 4 to 6 years

RUBEOLA (MEASLES): What is the risk for a child of developing pneumonia, encephalitis (inflammation of the brain), or degenerative disease of the nervous system with convulsions (subacute sclerosing panencephalitis) related to rubeola? The death rate for measles is .03 in 100,000.[27] Since 1984, over 55 percent of documented, confirmed cases of measles have been in fully immunized persons.[28] The greatest risk of the measles vaccine may be to push the incidence of this disease into the late teens and adulthood, when it is more likely to be fatal or cause more adverse and long-term effects.[29] The measles vaccine is a live vaccine and carries the risk that it will cause the patient to contract measles. Other adverse reactions include stinging or burning at the injection site, anaphylaxis, fever up to one month following injection, rash, cough, rhinitis, erythema multiforme, lymphadenopathy, urticaria, diarrhea, febrile convulsions, seizures, thrombocytopenia purpura, vasculitis, optic neuritis, retrobulbar neuritis, papillitis, retinitis, encephalitis and encephalopathy, ocular palsies, Guillain-Barré Syndrome, ataxia, and subacute sclerosing panencephalitis.[30] Measles vaccine is most often given as a part of the MMR, which includes the following side effects: burning or stinging at injection site, malaise, sore throat, cough, rhinitis, headache, dizziness, fever, rash, nausea, vomiting, diarrhea, induration, tenderness, lymphadenopathy, parotiditis, orchitis, nerve deafness, thrombocytopenia purpura, allergic reactions, urticaria, polyneuritis, arthralgia, arthritis, anaphylaxis, vasculitis, otitis media, conjunctivitis, febrile convulsions, seizures, syncope, erythema multiforme, optic neuritis, retrobulbar neuritis, papillitis, retinitis, encephalitis and encephalopathy, ocular palsies, Guillain-Barré Syndrome, ataxia, subacute sclerosing panencephalitis,[31] and a recent study from Europe indicates that there may be a link between the MMR (measles/mumps/rubella) vaccine and autism and irritable bowel syndrome.[32]

Measles vaccine contains chick embryo cells, neomycin, sorbitol, and hydrolyzed gelatin. MMR contains all live vaccines, chick embryo, cells from aborted babies, neomycin, sorbitol, and hydrolyzed gelatin.[33]

MUMPS: It is known that inflammation of the testicles, joints, kidneys, and/or thyroid, and hearing impairment related to mumps is rarely harmful in childhood, and that most of the above risks occur when mumps is contracted in adolescence or adulthood.[34]

The mumps vaccine poses the following risks: contraction of mumps from the live vaccine, burning or stinging at the injection site, anaphylaxis, cough, rhinitis, fever, diarrhea, vasculitis, parotiditis, orchitis, purpura, urticaria, erythema multiforme, optic neuritis, retrobulbar neuritis, syncope, encephalitis, febrile seizures, and nerve deafness.[35] Mumps is usually given in the MMR and may cause those side effects and adverse reactions as noted in the measles section above.

Mumps vaccine is live and should not be given to pregnant women. It is cultured in chick embryos and contains sorbitol and hydrolyzed gelatin.[36]

RUBELLA (GERMAN MEASLES): What is the risk for a child of developing inflammation of the brain or joints, and what is the risk of birth defects (including eye defects, heart defects, deafness, mental retardation, growth failure, jaundice, and disorders of blood clotting) in infants born to mothers who contract rubella during pregnancy, related to rubella? The greatest risk to a female may be if she never contracts rubella as a child but later when she is pregnant, causing damage to her unborn child. If she contracts rubella in childhood, she is immune for life, and prior to the vaccine 85 percent of the population was immune.[37] I understand that if a female is not immune as an adult, she can choose to take the vaccine prior to becoming pregnant. Many of those who contract rubella have been immunized (up to 80 percent).[38] Adverse reactions from the vaccine among teenage girls is 5 to 10 percent, and adverse reaction is 30 percent in adult women.[39] Adverse reactions include contracting rubella from the live virus in the vaccine, burning or stinging at the site, lymphadenopathy, urticaria, rash, malaise, sore throat, fever, headache, dizziness, nausea, vomiting, diarrhea, polyneuritis, arthralgia, arthritis, local pain and inflammation, erythema multiforme, cough, rhinitis, vasculitis, anaphylaxis, syncope, optic neuritis, retrobulbar neuritis, papillitis, Guillain-Barré Syndrome, encephalitis, thrombocytopenia purpura, and Chronic Fatigue Syndrome.[40] Rubella is most often administered in the MMR and may cause those side effects and adverse reactions listed under measles.

Rubella is cultured on the tissue of an aborted fetus. This child was the 27th child aborted and tested by researchers due to exposure to rubella in a pregnant woman. It contains neomycin, sorbitol, and hydrolyzed gelatin.[41]

HEPATITIS B Vaccine:
1. First dose at birth to 2 months
2. Second dose at 1 to 4 months
3. Third dose at 6 to 18 months

HEPATITIS B: What is the risk of a child developing hepatitis B viral infection, which can cause chronic inflammation of the liver leading to cirrhosis, liver cancer, and possibly death? The risk of developing hepatitis B is low if the mother is not a carrier or infected and if a child does not engage in promiscuous sex or use drugs. With antibiotic treatment for Hep B, most of those who contract it recover.[42] The Hep B vaccine only contains strains of Hep B and is not effective against Hep A, C, D, E, F, or G. The Hep B vaccine has the following reported side effects and adverse reactions: induration, erythema, swelling, fever, headache, dizziness, pain, pruritus, ecchymosis, sweating, malaise, chills, weakness, flushing, tingling, hypotension, flu-like symptoms, upper respiratory illness, nausea, anorexia, abdominal pain and cramping, vomiting, constipation, diarrhea, lymphadenopathy, pain or stiffness in muscles and joints, arthralgia, myalgia, back pain, rash, urticaria, petechiae, sleepiness, insomnia, irritability, agitation, anaphylaxis, angioedema, arthritis, tachycardia/palpitations, bronchospasm, abnormal liver function tests, dyspepsia, migraine, syncope, paresis neuropathy, hypothesis, paresthesis, Guillain-Barré Syndrome, Bell's Palsy, transverse myelitis, optic neuritis, multiple sclerosis, thrombocytopenia purpura, herpes zoster, alopecia, conjunctivitis, erythema nodosum, visual disturbances, vertigo, tinnitus, earache, and dysuria.[43] The studies only followed patients for four days post-vaccination.

The most commonly used Hep B vaccine contains thimerosal, although a relatively new release does not contain thimerosal. The vaccine also contains aluminum hydroxide, yeast protein, and phosphate buffers.[44]

VARICELLA (CHICKENPOX) Vaccine:
1. First dose at 12 to 18 months

VARICELLA (CHICKENPOX): What is the risk of a child developing chickenpox, which could potentially result in pneumonia, secondary skin or generalized infections, or, if caught during pregnancy, birth defects in the baby? It is understood that chickenpox is generally benign in children but results in an insignificant loss of hours at work for parents. Chickenpox in adults often manifests as shingles, a chronic and painful condition. It is known that contracting chickenpox later in life may increase the risk for herpes simplex. Side effects and adverse reactions for the chickenpox vaccine include contracting chickenpox from the live vaccine (27 percent), pain and redness at site, swelling, erythema, rash, pruritus, hematoma, induration, stiffness, upper respiratory illness, cough, irritability/nervousness, fatigue, disturbed sleep, diarrhea, loss of appetite, vomiting, otitis, diaper rash/contact rash, nausea, eye complaints, chills, lymphadenopathy, myalgia, lower respiratory illness, headache, teething, malaise, abdominal pain, other rash, allergic reactions including rash and hives, stiff neck, heat rash/prickly heat, arthralgia, eczema/dry skin/dermatitis, constipation, itching, pneumonitis, febrile seizures, and cold/canker sore.[45]

Varicella vaccine is cultured on cells from aborted babies and guinea pig cell cultures. It contains live virus, monosodium glutamate (MSG), sucrose, phosphate, processed gelatin, neomycin, and fetal calf serum.[46]

HEPATITIS A (HAV) Vaccine:
1. Two doses at least 6 months apart. Recommended in selected areas for children over 2 years of age.

HEPATITIS A (HAV): What is the risk of a child developing HAV, which could potentially result in prolonged or relapsed hepatitis, but will not result in chronic hepatitis disease?[47] HAV usually causes mild "flu-like" illness, jaundice, severe stomach pains and diarrhea, and, in rare cases, may result in death. Infection confers lifelong immunity.[48] The CDC admits that good personal hygiene (hand washing) and proper sanitation can prevent HAV.[49] HAV infection is spread by contaminated water or food, infected food handlers, unsanitary conditions following natural disasters, ingestion of raw or undercooked shellfish, institutionalized individuals, children not yet toilet trained, blood transfusions, or sharing needles with infected people. Transmission is most likely in developing countries where sanitation is poor and infection rate of children under 5 is 90 percent before they reach that age. Fatality rate is less than .6 percent overall, and 70 percent of those deaths occur in patients over 49 years, many of whom have underlying liver disease.[50] Other at-risk populations include those living on American Indian reservations and in Alaskan Native villages, homosexually active men, IV drug users, people using clotting factor concentrates, and international travelers.[51] Side effects and adverse reactions from the vaccine include injection-site soreness, headache, fever, malaise, induration, redness, swelling, fatigue, anorexia, nausea, pruritus, rash, urticaria, pharyngitis, upper respiratory tract infections, abdominal pain, diarrhea, dysgeusia, vomiting, arthralgia, elevated creatine phosphokinase, myalgia, lymphadenopathy, hypertonic episodes, insomnia, photophobia, and vertigo.[52]

Aborted fetal tissue is an ingredient in the Havrix Hep A vaccine, as is formaldehyde, aluminum hydroxide, and 2-phenoxyethanol.[53] *There is currently a combination Hep A and B vaccine, Twinrix, being tested in the UK.*[54] *Twinrix is grown in human cell cultures, contains 2-phenoxyethanol, neomycin sulfate, polysorbate, tromentamol, and formaldehyde.*[55]

PNEUMOCOCCAL Vaccine:
1. First dose at 2 months
2. Second dose at 4 months
3. Third dose at 6 months
4. Fourth dose at 12 to 18 months

PNEUMOCOCCAL: What is the risk for children of developing pneumococcal disease, which could result in meningitis, blood infection, pneumonia, and/or ear infections? Studies indicate that this vaccine may only decrease ear infections by 9 percent, and may only result in a 20 percent reduction in chronic ear infections and ear tube insertion in that group. A child has a 7.5 in 5,000 chance of developing this disease if he or she is under age 2 and a 1 in 5,000 chance of developing it if over age 2. Risk factors for developing this disease are immunoglobulin deficiency, nephrotic syndrome, Hodgkin's disease, congenital or acquired immunodeficiency, some upper respiratory infections, splenic dysfunctions, splenectomy, or organ transplant. This vaccine (PCV) was originally marketed for immunocompromised children.[56] This vaccine is contraindicated in children with thrombocytopenia, coagulation disorders, or sensitivity to diphtheria toxoid.[57] Possible side effects and complications from the vaccine include erythema, induration, tenderness, interference of limb movement, inflammation, fever, irritability, drowsiness, restless sleep, decreased appetite, vomiting, diarrhea, fussiness, rash, hives, bronchitis, asthma, pneumonia, otitis media (ear infection), sepsis, seizure, anaphylaxis, and death.[58] Recipients were followed for three days and almost 10 percent of the subjects made a visit to the emergency room in the follow-up period. There were eight cases of SIDS in the 17,066 subjects involved in the trial.[59] Note: Children in the study's control group received another experimental vaccine, so there have been no trial studies done with children who received no vaccine.[60]

Prevnar contains .125 mg of aluminum sulfate, protein polysaccharides from seven strains of strep. pneumonia bacteria, diphtheria toxin, casamino acids, yeast extract. Studies indicate that it may interfere with the safety and efficacy of other vaccines.[61]

ROTAVIRUS Vaccine:
1. First dose at 2 months
2. Second dose at 4 months
3. Third dose at 6 months

ROTAVIRUS: What is the risk of an infant or young child developing a severe acute gastroenteritis from a rotavirus leading to severe diarrhea, acute dehydration, and intussusception (a serious and life-threatening event that occurs when a part of the intestine gets blocked or twisted)? Studies show that over 600,000 children under 5 years of age are affected by this virus in developing countries[62] and over 50,000 are hospitalized in the United States each year.[63] Epidemiologists acknowledge that incidence of infection has decreased significantly due to improvement in sanitation and nutrition, water quality, zinc, breastfeeding, hygiene, and the availability of oral rehydration solution (ORS). The primary mode of transmission is the fecal-oral route. Children not exposed to the daycare setting are seldom affected.

RotaShield was the name of the first rotavirus vaccine developed. It was recalled in 1999 after being attributed to intestinal twisting in young children. This first vaccine demonstrated an incidence of intussusception that was 30 times greater than normal.[64] The newest version, RotaTeq, came out in 2006, and has been added to the recommended childhood immunization schedule. RotaTeq contains five live viruses that replicate in the small intestine; four are isolated from humans and one from a bovine (cow) host. Despite not being adequately tested before its release, over 3.5 million doses of the new vaccine have been given to children. The shot is injected in a three-time series to young infants and toddlers. There have been reports of stomach conditions as adverse reactions, but none that have caused the FDA to look into it until recently. Over 28 cases of infants and toddlers needing intestinal surgery after receiving the RotaTeq vaccine prompted the latest warning. While it is not yet enough to recall the vaccine and pull it off the shelves, it has prompted a CDC investigation.

The most common side effects reported after taking RotaTeq were diarrhea, vomiting, fever, runny nose and sore throat, wheezing or coughing, and ear infection. In some cases where intestinal twisting has occurred, the fact that all these young children were recently vaccinated for rotavirus is a huge cause for concern and is quite likely directly related.[65]

HUMAN PAPILLOMAVIRUS (HPV) Vaccine:

At the time of publication, the HPV vaccine, Gardasil, has been approved for use by the FDA. However, it has only been mandated by the state of Texas, which prompted concern and legislative debate. Presently, the citizens of Texas are using their right of exemption to avoid the governor's mandate. In two other states (Virginia and New Jersey), legislation is pending.

HUMAN PAPILLOMAVIRUS (HPV): What is the risk of females developing genital warts or cervical cancer as a result of infection with this virus? It is understood that about 20 million people in the United States are infected with HPV, and by age 50 at least 80 percent of women will have had an HPV infection. According to the Centers for Disease Control, most women exposed to the virus do not develop genital warts or cervical cancer. HPV is a common virus spread by sex. There are 127 strains of the HPV, only four of which were targeted for the vaccine, HPV-6, HPV-11, HPV-16, and HPV-18. Strains of HPV-16 and HPV-18 account for 70 percent of cervical cancers, and HPV-6 and HPV-11 account for about 90 percent of genital warts. Without any attempt to minimize the seriousness of cervical cancer, statistics show that just 3,719 women died of cervical cancer in one year, compared to heart disease, which kills over 300,000 annually. The vaccine targets primarily 11- to 12-year-old girls, who are not usually sexually active.[66] Men and boys are affected by genital warts, but no research is available to determine the rate.

The vaccine Gardasil was developed for the four HPV strains mentioned above. The FDA approved the vaccine in mid-2006. A five-year study by Merck, the vaccine maker, tested 25,000 women in third world countries; 1,184 were pre-teen girls, but no data was provided that is specific to this age group. According to British medical journal *The Lancet*, the vaccine is only effective for four and one-half years. A booster will be needed in five years, though to date no long-term studies have been done. The effectiveness or dangers of this vaccine will not be known for at least a decade.

Common side effects were soreness at site of injection, dizziness, temporary paralysis, and loss of speech (as reported to the Vaccine Adverse Events Reporting System). Since approval of the vaccine in June 2006, there have been 1,261 adverse reports.[67] This vaccine is highly controversial since so little is known about it and its ramifications for the future.

Adult Immunization Schedule (BIG SHOTS)

The same adverse reactions, side effects, and risk factors exist for children (BABY SHOTS) and adults (BIG SHOTS) receiving conventional vaccinations. In addition, many adults are advised to have a flu shot annually.

ANNUAL FLU VACCINE: The flu shot, given each year especially to the elderly, is not without problems. This vaccine contains formaldehyde, a known cancer-causing agent. It also contains the preservative thimerosal, a derivative of mercury that is a known neurotoxin linked to brain damage and autoimmune diseases. Aluminum is yet another flu vaccine ingredient. Mercury and aluminum are two toxic heavy metals that have been associated with an increased incidence of Alzheimer's disease.

Adverse reactions reported as a result of the annual flu vaccine include allergic asthma, fever, hives, general malaise, muscle pain, respiratory tract infections, gastrointestinal problems, eye problems, abnormal blood pressure, and other circulatory abnormalities. Moreover, those with a severe allergy to eggs are advised against the flu shot because the flu vaccine is propagated on chicken/duck embryo cells.

Influenza A and B are the main two virus strains detected during the flu season. But there are many strains of influenza viruses, and, moreover, existing strains mutate all the time. It is, therefore, an extremely difficult task to foresee the causative agent of a new influenza epidemic and even more difficult to produce a corresponding vaccine in time for it to be effective. The constant mutation of the viruses—and the unpredictability of which virus to use—makes the whole influenza vaccination business a game of roulette. The actual composition of the flu vaccine is based on an educated guess made by a consensus of about thirty public-health experts. These experts meet annually with the FDA in the U.S. to predict which specific strains of influenza will invade the country in the coming year. Therefore, the effectiveness of the flu vaccine is less than 20 percent.

It is interesting to note that influenza outbreaks still occur despite widespread use of the recommended flu vaccine. The reason given for such immunization failures is that the wrong virus was predicted for use in the flu vaccine.

Vaccination proponents are at a loss to explain such figures. They are also at a loss to explain why it is that so many unvaccinated individuals do not get the flu. I would suggest that it has to do with an individual's immune system.

A healthy immune system is a strong defense against disease. Even if you or your child have been vaccinated by the conventional route, there is a great deal you can and ought to do to enhance the immune system naturally. There are no magic bullets that will guarantee freedom from infectious illness. However, your immunity and therefore your resistance to infectious disease can be greatly improved by following the basic diet and lifestyle guidelines outlined in this book.

Part II

The Action Plan

Chapter 3

Developing Immunity: There Are Alternatives

Our immune system is a comprehensive, multi-faceted, and un-believably sophisticated system by which our bodies are able to naturally resist disease and infection. It fights off invading bacteria, viruses, and other organisms that surround us constantly in our potentially hostile environment.

The most important ways to increase immunity are also the most simple. Parents, children, and travelers can enhance the body's natural immune system and make it as strong as possible with proper diet, exercise, and common-sense choices. These will contribute to the body's defense system to ward off and fight many illnesses, such as the common cold and flu. Even more complex illnesses, such as rheumatoid arthritis and diphtheria, can be controlled or defeated by the immunity our bodies can develop. This process begins before the child is born.

Breastfeeding: Nutritional Benefits

Human milk is the best food for babies. A living, biological fluid, breast milk contains the right amount of nutrients—in the right proportions—for the growing baby. For example, lactoferrin provides optimal absorption of iron and protects the gut from harmful bacteria; lipases assist in digestion of fats; and special growth factors and hormones contribute to optimal growth and development. Mother's milk changes during a feeding from thirst-quenching to hunger-satisfying, and it comes in a variety of flavors reflecting the diversity of the mother's diet. Its composition changes as the baby grows to meet baby's changing nutritional needs. It serves as the nutritional model for artificial baby milks, but none of these can match it. While most people are aware that human milk provides excellent nutrition that assists the developing immune system, many people are unaware of breastfeeding's other health benefits for babies.

Breastfeeding and the Immune System

Human milk is a baby's first immunization. Many of the early benefits of breastfeeding are derived from colostrum. It is mammary fluid secreted the first few days after delivery. It is packed with components (such as antibodies and natural antibiotics) which increase immunity and protect the newborn's intestines against bacteria and viruses. It also provides essential nutrients, including growth factors, vitamins, minerals, and hormones. It is important that colostrum should be derived from human milk and not animal sources.

Artificially fed babies have higher rates of middle ear infections, pneumonia, and gastroenteritis (stomach flu). Breastfeeding protects the developing immune system from cancers such as lymphoma, bowel diseases such as Crohn's disease and celiac sprue, and juvenile rheumatoid arthritis, all of which are related to immune system function. Also, breastfed babies generally mount a more effective response to childhood immunizations. In all these cases, benefits begin immediately and increase with extended duration of breastfeeding.

Babies from families with a tendency to allergic diseases particularly benefit from breastfeeding. Exclusive breastfeeding, especially if it continues for at least six months, provides protection against allergies, asthma, eczema, infections, and disease.

UNICEF has long encouraged breastfeeding for two years and longer, and the American Academy of Pediatrics is now on record as encouraging mothers to nurse at least one year and as long after as both mother and baby desire. Breastfeeding until age three or four was common in much of the world until recently, and it is still common in many societies for toddlers to breastfeed.

Immunity can be enhanced, and food allergies can be minimized or prevented, if solid foods and beverages are introduced to the breastfed infant properly. High-protein and highly allergenic foods should be introduced, ideally, after 21 months of age. These include citrus, chocolate, wheat, corn, nuts, and foods containing yeast. It is my opinion that cow's milk, eggs, and other high-protein animal products should not be introduced at all. For non-animal products, it is best to introduce one new food at a time every four days, noting such reactions as sneezing, runny nose, rash, irritability, diarrhea, or vomiting. If a food causes any of these reactions, it should be avoided. Ideally, well-tolerated foods should be rotated on a four-day basis so as to minimize sensitization that often occurs when foods are eaten repetitively.

A Safe Environment for the Maturing Immune System

Children attending daycare centers are very good at sharing a number of bacterial, viral, and parasitic infections with each other. Daycare is an ideal environment for the spread of disease because the children move about and interact with each other, their personal hygiene is less than ideal, their ability to control their bodily secretions and excretions is poor, and their immune systems are not yet fully developed. These are age-related risk factors that continue to exist even in kindergarten, preschool, and elementary school.

- The Fecal-Oral Route: This is responsible for *Escherichia coli* O157:H7, hepatitis A, rotavirus, and salmonella infections. Note that the risk for food contamination is higher when the person who prepares or serves the food also changes the children's diapers.
- The Respiratory Route: This is responsible for Bordetella pertussis, Haemophilus influenzae, pneumococcal, Mycobacterium tuberculosis, Streptococcus pneumonia, measles, mumps, and varicella zoster virus infections.
- By Skin Contact: This is responsible for head lice and scabies infections.
- Blood, Urine, or Saliva Routes: They are responsible for cytomegalovirus, hepatitis B and C virus, and herpes simplex virus infections.

Many parents and guardians choose homeschool options to avoid the potential risks that exist in the environment of daycare centers and elementary schools. Immunity depends largely on what individuals do to strengthen the immune system and protect the body.

Chapter 4

Optimizing the System: IMMUNITY

A Lifestyle Approach

We want to feel alive and energetic, look forward to each day, and enjoy optimum health. To experience this, each of us must assume responsibility in an intelligent way for our own well-being and that of our families; yet, we do not have the years of training and experience needed to be a physician. What can we do to take charge of our health?

Try IMMUNITY, an easy way to remember the building blocks of healthful living. This program is based upon the eight relatively simple concepts that have been proven to improve your health, decrease your risk of disease, and strengthen your body's immunity. These simple principles provide the foundation for dealing with any health condition successfully. IMMUNITY stands for

Ions/**Fresh Air**

Moderation/**Temperance**

Movement/**Exercise**

Ultraviolet B/**Sunshine**

Nutrition

Immersion in **Water**

Trust in **Divine Power**

Yearning for **Rest**

Applied individually, each health principle is very effective; combined, the benefits are multiplied far in excess of what each one by itself could do.

IONS/FRESH AIR

The body and mind must have oxygen to survive, yet most people take the air they breathe for granted. Since the beginning of the industrial revolution, air pollution has increased dramatically. Indoors we face accumulated air pollution from such varied sources as tobacco smoke; formaldehyde from wood products; chemical fumes from copy machines, carpeting, upholstery, and cleaning products; carbon monoxide and nitrogen dioxide from heating appliances that burn coal, oil, gas, wood, and kerosene; as well as dust, mold, insect droppings, fungi, ozone, lead, asbestos, pesticides, and radon gas. Symptoms of these pollutants include sore throats, coughing, burning eyes, headaches, sluggishness, nausea, dizziness, exhaustion, and depression. This cluster of symptoms is often referred to as "sick building syndrome." You can protect yourself by limiting your exposure to these pollutants and bringing in fresh air to ventilate the indoors.

Fresh air, especially that found in natural settings around trees and moving water, in sunlight, and after thunderstorms, is chemically different from the indoor air most of us breathe. This ionized, electrically charged air has been proven to benefit the health. It improves the brain's ability to function by clarifying the mind, improving concentration, and boosting learning abilities. Fresh air brings a sense of happiness and well-being by altering brain levels of serotonin. It improves sleep quality and kills bacteria and viruses in the air. Pollution causes air to lose these capabilities.

Devitalized air increases tension, anxiety, lethargy, and irritability. It is linked with increased asthma, other respiratory problems, and headaches. Do your utmost to get as much fresh air as you can every day. If possible, move to a more rural setting. Indoor plants can help to purify the air, and a city park provides at least some trees and plants to improve air quality. Taking several slow, deep breaths gives you a shot of oxygen and helps the body unload carbon dioxide. Daily exercise helps you to breathe deeply, which saturates your body with oxygen. If you are fighting sickness, get as much fresh air as possible. In combination with the other principles of health, it is a powerful remedy.

MODERATION/TEMPERANCE

The word *temperance*, when used in the context of health, has three very distinct meanings: moderation in the use of that which is good, total abstinence from that which is harmful, and self-restraint.

More is not always better. Work, exercise, rest, eating, and sunshine are all important and necessary, but any of them taken to extremes becomes harmful. Overeating, even of the healthiest foods, is harmful. Exercise is indispensable to living healthfully, but too much causes injury.

It is counterproductive to good health to do anything that harms the body. Avoid tobacco, alcohol, drugs, and caffeinated drinks. Do not use fat, salt, protein, or sugar to excess. Avoid things that are harmful to you personally: foods to which you are sensitive or which contribute to a disease you are fighting, risky behaviors or activities, certain people or thought patterns, and so on. The rule simply stated: "First, do no harm."

This is easily said, but self-restraint is an elusive creature for most of us. It is sobering and alarming to realize that often we are not really in control of ourselves, that we are slaves to some appetite or habit. If you find that you do not have the power to accomplish what you choose, there is hope. Read this entire chapter, especially the section on Trust in Divine Power.

MOVEMENT/EXERCISE

We are created for action, and it is impossible to be truly well without it. The adage "use it or lose it" applies to every part of the body. Yet, for many, the greatest exertion of the day is getting out of bed or walking from the kitchen to the garage. Now we must deliberately incorporate physical activity into our lives. Exercise is of critical importance in a total-lifestyle approach to health. Some benefits of exercise:

- Exercise helps us feel good. It is so effective that it is a valuable tool for fighting depression and relieving anxiety and stress.
- Exercise increases energy levels, impacting efficiency and productivity in the other areas of life.
- Exercise helps one to reach and maintain proper weight. It burns calories, builds muscle, and increases the metabolism.
- Exercise greatly strengthens the immune system. This reduces not only cold and flu infections but also significantly reduces cancer mortality rates.[68]
- Exercise enhances circulation, which in turn improves memory and mental ability, gives better sleep, and promotes faster healing. It decreases the pain and stiffness of osteoarthritis by delivering blood to the joints, and it also relieves tension headaches.
- Exercise strengthens the bones, helping them retain calcium and other minerals, thus preventing osteoporosis.

- Exercise protects from heart disease by strengthening the heart, decreasing blood pressure and heart rate, and lowering LDL (bad) cholesterol while raising HDL (good) cholesterol.
- Exercise aids digestion and promotes intestinal activity by reducing gas and constipation.

Exercise Essentials

- Check with your doctor before starting a *vigorous* exercise program if you have cardiovascular disease or are over 40 with multiple cardiovascular risk factors. The risks of physical activity are very low compared to the health benefits. More people rust out than wear out.
- Make physical activity a part of your life: grow a garden; when possible, choose to walk rather than ride; always use the most distant parking space; take the stairs.
- Play active games with the kids; use a push mower; walk the dog. In addition to these activities, choose an exercise that you will enjoy such as walking, swimming, or cycling. This cannot be stressed enough: if you don't enjoy it, you won't make it a permanent part of your life.
- Pick a time of day that's best for you and keep that exercise appointment as if it were a business engagement. Exercise is cumulative. Three 10-minute sessions are just as good as one 30-minute period.
- Always start with a low-intensity exercise to let your body warm up. Then do a few stretching exercises using slow, steady movements.
- End with a low-intensity exercise to cool down, and do some more stretching to avoid soreness and enhance flexibility.

Walking

One of the simplest exercises is walking. Invest in a good pair of walking shoes and dress appropriately for the weather. Some surprising advantages of walking:

- Walking uses almost all of the body's 206 bones and 640 muscles.
- It is something that almost everyone can do without learning new skills.
- It is easy on the joints.
- It does not require expensive equipment.
- The pace is easy to adjust.
- It can be done anywhere, from shopping malls to the great outdoors.
- Walking especially lends itself to socializing. People make exercise fun, so include friends and family members. If they won't join you, take the dog.

- You need at least 30 minutes of exercise every day. If daily exercise is not possible, try for three times a week on non-consecutive days. Alternating aerobic exercise with strength training is now recommended as the most complete and beneficial program.
- Remember, you aren't in competition with anyone, so don't push beyond your tolerance. Excessive exercise is not healthy.

ULTRAVIOLET B/SUNSHINE

Sunshine has gotten some bad publicity recently; the impression has been given that even small amounts of sun are harmful. While it is true that excessive sunlight can increase the risk of skin cancer and cataracts, sunshine in judicious amounts is extremely beneficial.

- Sunlight converts cholesterol into vitamin D, lowering the blood cholesterol. Vitamin D provides a host of benefits to the body, including prevention of many types of cancer and better calcium absorption, which in turn helps prevent osteoporosis and tooth decay, makes stronger bones, and speeds bone repair.
- Sunlight kills germs and enhances the immune system by increasing the oxygen capacity of the red blood cells and increasing gamma globulin. It also raises the number and effectiveness of the white blood cells, which destroy both germs and cancerous cells. Lightly tanned skin kills germs and resists infection much better than untanned skin. Many skin diseases respond well to controlled doses of sunlight.
- Sunlight benefits the nervous system and is important in treating depression. It gives a sense of well-being by increasing endorphin production in the brain.
- Sunlight benefits the cardiovascular system. It improves the circulation, lowers the heart rate, and normalizes the blood pressure and blood sugar, bringing highs down and lows up. Sunlight aids in weight loss, increasing the metabolism by stimulating thyroid production.
- Sunlight improves sleep. Natural light exposure in daytime increases melatonin output at night.
- Sunlight enhances waste elimination by improving liver function; for example, it is an effective treatment for jaundice. It relieves the kidneys of some of their burden by eliminating wastes through the skin when you sweat.

Moderate work or exercise outdoors every day will secure these benefits and more. Sunlight still reaches us on cloudy days, but glass filters out 95 percent of the beneficial ultraviolet rays.

Skin Cancer
Sun should be taken in moderation. Overexposure to sunlight is a major risk factor for skin cancer. Melanoma, a quick-spreading skin cancer that is fatal in 20 percent of cases, is caused by repeated burning of the skin. Avoid sunburn like the plague. Get your sunshine in small doses and take great care between 10 a.m. and 3 p.m., when the sun is strongest. Moderate sunshine provides so many benefits that avoiding sunlight altogether is not a healthy choice.

NUTRITION
How would you like to enjoy tasty, satisfying meals, normalize your weight, and enhance your health all at the same time? It is possible! Many absolutely delicious foods are both healthful and enjoyable.

Food is vitally important to our health. It provides the raw material for growth and repair and also provides the fuel for our bodies to function. It is a key element in the length and quality of life. Poor diet contributes to weight gain, heart disease, cancer, and a host of other diseases.

Understanding Food
The basic components of food are carbohydrates, proteins, and fats. Other components include fiber, micronutrients, and phytochemicals.

Carbohydrates: These are the primary source of energy for every action and process in the body. Carbohydrates come in two forms: sugar and starch. Sugars are digested very quickly and, unless fiber is present to slow things down, enter the blood stream as glucose within minutes. Starches take longer to digest and provide energy for a longer period of time. They should constitute the largest percentage of the diet, but pay attention to where they come from. When foods are refined, the fiber is removed. This results in a denser concentration of calories, making it easier to eat more than you can use. These excess calories are converted to fat and stored. Whole grains, potatoes, beans, vegetables, and fruit are all excellent sources of carbohydrates.

Proteins: Your body is built largely of protein. It is the most important component of muscles, blood, skin, bones, nails, hair, and the internal organs. It is necessary for the growth, maintenance, and repair of the body. Protein takes longer to digest than starch. It is broken down by the digestive system into amino acids, which the body then uses to build its own proteins. Ideally protein should make up no more than 12 percent of the diet. Excess protein is changed to uric acid and eliminated, or it is converted to glucose and used for fuel. Good sources of protein are beans, grains, and vegetables.

Fat: This is necessary for the proper functioning of the body, especially the brain. Fat regulates many body functions, helps to absorb certain vitamins, makes food taste good, and gives a feeling of satisfaction. It is the most difficult nutrient for the digestive system to handle and takes three to four hours to digest. It should comprise no more than 15 percent of the diet. For the vegetarian, this breaks down to 4 percent saturated fat, 6 percent monounsaturated fat, and 5 percent polyunsaturated fat each day. In order to comply with this recommendation, use oils high in omega-3 fats, such as olive oil, walnut, flaxseed, and other nut oils. Excess fat is simply stored to be used as a backup source of fuel. High-fat foods include meat and dairy products, nuts, and "free fats"—refined fats from which all other nutrients are removed. Low-fat foods include beans, grains, vegetables, and fruit.

Fiber: While it contributes no nutrients, fiber fills you up, thus limiting calorie intake. It slows down the digestion of sugar, helping to keep blood sugar levels stable; in addition, it speeds up the time it takes food to move through the digestive system, which keeps it from decaying before it is eliminated. A diet based on unrefined plant foods contains enough fiber to properly regulate the digestive system.

Micronutrients: Vitamins, minerals, and other micronutrients are substances the body needs in small amounts to work properly and stay healthy. It has been proven that a diet of pure carbohydrates, protein, and fat without the micronutrients will result in death. When foods are refined, the majority of both vitamins and minerals are removed. For instance, when wheat is refined to make white flour, 24 vitamins and minerals are lost; when it is "enriched," four or five of the lost micronutrients are replaced.

Phytochemicals: These are literally "plant chemicals." They are various substances found in plants that demonstrably lower the risk of cancer. Most work by either blocking cancer-causing agents from affecting the cells or by suppressing malignant body cells to keep them from growing. Phytochemicals are usually destroyed when foods are refined.

A Diet of Excess

Most of the diseases that plague our society today, including heart disease, hypertension, cancer, osteoporosis, and diabetes, are closely connected to our dietary habits. The typical American meal is high in fat, protein, and refined carbohydrates, such as sugar and white flour, and low in unrefined carbohydrates, such as natural fruits, grains, and vegetables.

In the past hundred years the incidence of heart disease and stroke has risen from 15 percent to 45 percent of all causes of death. Cancer has risen from 6 percent to 25 percent of all causes. This rise in disease is directly related to diet. Countries in which the people do not have access to a Western diet have a much lower incidence of these diseases.

Americans are dying from a diet of excess: too much fat, too much protein, too much cholesterol, too much sugar, and too much salt. We eat too many calories and we eat too often. Some of the problems:

Fat

Most people don't realize that they are consuming an average of 37 percent of their daily calories as fat. This is much more than the body can properly handle. Excess fat is a major contributor to heart disease, cancer, diabetes, and poor self-image.

Protein

Respected nutritional scientist Dr. Mark Messina, formerly of the National Cancer Institute's Diet and Cancer branch, sums it up. He says that "when people eat several servings of grains, beans, and vegetables throughout the day and get enough calories, it is virtually impossible to be deficient in protein."[69] Rather than most people getting too little protein, Westerners eat two to three times more than they need. Excess protein in the body leaches calcium from the bones and is a major contributor to osteoporosis. In one study men on low- (48g), medium- (95g), and high- (142g) protein diets were given 1,400 mg of calcium per day for four months. The low-protein group gained 20 mg of calcium per day. The medium-protein group lost 30mg of calcium per day, and the high-protein group lost 70 mg of calcium per day.[70] Too much protein also causes deterioration of kidney function and is linked to increased risk of cancer. Research and epidemiological studies correlate high protein intake with increased growth rates and decreased life span.

Salt

We eat 10 to 20 times more salt than is needed. Salt contributes prominently to high blood pressure, heart failure, and kidney disease. The body only needs about one tenth of a teaspoon (½ gram) of salt a day. However, that drastic a change is unrealistic for most people. A more reasonable goal is to cut back from two to four teaspoons (10 to 20 grams) a day to one teaspoon (5 grams) per day.

Sugar

Devoid of fiber and nutrients, refined sugars are empty calories that account for up to 20 percent of daily caloric intake for many people. Sugars produce a quick rise in blood sugar and energy. They cause the body to overreact and flood the system with insulin, which drops the blood sugar too fast and too far, causing low blood sugar and an energy dip, often accompanied by a feeling of faintness and hunger. Jumping through the day from "sugar high" to "the sugar blues" is a way of life for many people.

Empty Calories

Many beverages such as soda, beer, sweetened coffee and tea, and other drinks are loaded with calories. These, along with high-sugar and high-fat snacks, not only add thousands of unnecessary calories but take the place of balanced, nutritious food, leaving you over-caloried and undernourished.

The original diet intended for man consisted of grains, fruits, nuts, and vegetables (Genesis 1:29, 3:18). Prepared as simply as possible, they are the most healthful and nourishing foods available. They give longevity, strength, endurance, intellectual acuity, and freedom from disease.

Putting it all together

Here is a practical plan that provides a complete balance of essential nutrients for radiant good health:

- Eat a wide variety of fruits, grains, vegetables, legumes, seeds, and nuts prepared in a simple and tasty way. There are hundreds of varieties and colors in every imaginable texture, shape, and flavor. Eating a varied selection of natural plant foods will furnish all the fat, protein, fiber, and other nutrients the body needs. For maximum health and energy, the human body needs a low-fat, moderate-protein, high-carbohydrate diet.
- Avoid protein from animal sources, since animal products provide an excess of fat, cholesterol, and protein; they often carry harmful viruses and bacteria, as well as hormones, antibiotics, and other chemical concentrations. Bacteria and viruses in animal protein will expose the immune systems to infections.

- Limit fat, sugar, and salt. Choose naturally sweet foods such as dried fruit rather than refined sugar, and choose olives, nuts and avocados —all in moderation— rather than refined fats and oils.
- Eat a good breakfast, a moderate lunch, and a light supper two to three hours before bedtime, or skip the evening meal. A large breakfast containing a proper balance of nutrients will give you steady energy all morning. According to the notable Alameda County study, eating breakfast has almost as much of a positive impact on health and longevity as abstinence from tobacco.[71] Timing of food is an important factor in good health. Food eaten in the morning is used during the day. Food taken late in the day is stored as fat. Studies have shown that people have lost as much as 10 pounds a month merely by timing their meals correctly.[72] A heavy evening meal also increases the number of fat particles in your blood, setting you up for a heart attack while you sleep.
- Allow at least five hours between meals, and eat meals at the same time each day. This gives your digestive system the opportunity to work efficiently and rest between cycles.
- Don't eat between meals. This slows down digestion so that food in the stomach ferments and produces toxins. It normally takes four to five hours for food to leave the stomach after a meal. In one study a person was given snacks every hour and a half after breakfast. Thirteen hours later more than half of the breakfast was still undigested. Each time food is put into the stomach, it stops the digestion process, mixes everything up, and starts over.
- Beverages with calories should not be consumed between meals for the same reason; those calories interrupt the digestion as well.

How do we implement this nutritional plan? When you shop, choose fresh fruits and vegetables, wholegrain bread and pasta, low-sugar cereals, brown rice, raw nuts and seeds, dried fruit without sugar coating, and so on. If you buy prepared foods, read the labels and avoid foods high in fat, sugar, salt, and spices. Even some "health" foods may be high in these things. When you cook, avoid frying; boil, steam, or bake instead. Cook grains and beans well; cook fruits and vegetables lightly. While there are many good cookbooks available to help you with a vegetarian diet, it is best to just keep meals simple and uncomplicated. You don't have to be a gourmet chef to prepare appetizing meals.

Bear in mind, however, that our taste buds are very over-stimulated with the processed foods many of us are used to. It takes a little while to adjust to more simply prepared meals, so persevere. Tasting a new or different food 10 times is usually all it takes to retrain the taste buds.

However, forcing yourself to eat things you really cannot stand is counterproductive. Utilize the natural foods that you enjoy, but periodically go back and try some of the foods you've rejected — you may find that they become much more edible as your taste buds adjust.

Implement these changes one step at a time. Focus your efforts on what is most important to you, then as each new change becomes a habit, take the next step toward improving your nutrition. Finally, don't force the changes you make on others; just enjoy your new lifestyle until your friends and family desire the kind of radiant health which is now yours.

IMMERSION IN WATER

Water is to the body what oil is to a car engine. It is the universal lubricant that makes everything else work. The body loses 10 to 12 cups of water a day, which need to be replaced. The food we eat each day provides two to four cups of water, so we only need to drink about 6 to 8 glasses a day. When our bodies do not get sufficient water, the blood thickens, increasing the risk of stroke and heart disease. A lack of water dehydrates the red blood cells so they have a greater tendency to clot. Insufficient water can mimic hypoglycemia, causing headaches, tiredness, and fainting spells. One of the best things you can do to help your body when you are ill is to drink plenty of water. This replaces any fluid lost during a fever and insures that every part of your body will function well.

Other kinds of beverages cannot do what water does. A glass of water acts as a bath for the digestive system, cleansing and refreshing it. Soda and coffee can no more clean the inside of your body than they can the outside. Many beverages actually result in a loss of water from the system, meaning it requires more water to metabolize the sugar in the beverage than it can provide. Caffeine and alcohol are both diuretics which cause the body to lose water. You need an extra glass of water for every caffeinated or alcoholic beverage you drink.

Drinking water with meals dilutes the gastric juices and slows the digestive process. The best time to drink water is between meals, no less than fifteen minutes before eating or one hour afterwards.

Water on the Outside

A clean body and surroundings are indispensable for physical and mental health. Used externally, hot and cold water can help reduce swelling and pain, boost immunity, and bring comfort and relaxation.

Water (as steam, liquid, or ice) does an excellent job of radiating and absorbing heat. Ice makes things cold much faster than air of the same temperature, and warm water will warm your feet up much more quickly than if you held them close to a heater. Our bodies have a number of different reactions to heat and cold that can be used to effectively promote health and healing:

- Heat causes the blood vessels to expand, makes the immune system more effective, and decreases muscle pain and stiffness in arthritis. Prolonged mild heat soothes, sedates, and relieves muscle spasms.
- Cold causes the blood vessels to contract, decreases swelling and inflammation, and can decrease hemorrhage and muscle pain. Prolonged cold rapidly decreases the effectiveness of the immune system.
- The application of heat and cold through water can do wonders for conditions related to poor circulation and congestion, a condition where too much blood collects in one place. Increasing the circulation accelerates cell metabolism and speeds nutrient delivery and waste removal from the cells. Use water applications to strengthen the immune system and speed the healing process in a specific organ or member of the body. All types of arthritis respond well to improved circulation.

Alternate the application of hot and cold water to the entire body or to specific parts of it for these effects. The best effect is obtained by a ratio of about three minutes of hot to one minute of cold.

When too much blood accumulates in one part of the body, as in the case of tension headaches and menstrual cramps, the congestion can be relieved by putting the feet in hot water and applying a cold cloth to the congested area. This will draw more blood to the feet, relieving the pressure on the head or abdomen.

Caution: Diabetics and others with impaired feeling in the extremities, make sure the water is no hotter than 100° F. to avoid burns. For more information about water treatments, see the Appendix.

TRUST IN DIVINE POWER

What do faith, religion, and trust in God have to do with health? The list of benefits is extensive. Research has shown that spirituality helps to control stress, strengthen the immune system, and protect against heart disease and cancer. Beyond these scientifically verifiable benefits, God promises eternal life to those who trust Him—a life of perfect health and freedom from pain, fear, and death.

But can I trust Him? Does He even exist, and if so, does He care about me personally? Before you can trust a person—God or man—you have to get to know him, observe his personality and character, communicate and interact with him, consider how he treats others and whether he keeps his promises. Before you can trust God, you need to become acquainted, talk and listen to Him, work with Him, and investigate how He deals with His children. He longs to develop a close, personal relationship with you. He invites you to come to Him on a daily basis and learn of Him.

Listening to God

Ask God to give you spiritual insight so that you may hear and understand what He is saying to you. Here are some of the more common ways God speaks to us:

Through the life of Christ. God sent His son into the world so we might have a clearer picture of His personality and character. Christ's life of compassion, courtesy, and service to others here on this earth culminated in His death on the cross, the most vivid portrayal of God's love ever seen.

Through the Bible. This book is God's disclosure of His own character. He reveals the true story of the conflict between Himself and Satan and how it has played out through history.

Through nature. God created the wonderful and beautiful things of nature for the happiness and well-being of all His creatures. His love and wisdom can be seen in His created works. Though the earth bears evidence of the curse of sin and only dimly reflects the Creator's glory, His object lessons are not obliterated. Nature still speaks of her Creator. Imperfect and blighted though she may be, His craftsmanship may still be recognized.

Through others. Like the moon reflecting the light of the sun, Christians can give you a small glimpse of what God is like. However, the image of Christ in them may be partial, incomplete, or even distorted. It is better to look to the Source.

Through providence (God's personal care, protection, and guidance in your life). God intervenes in our lives. He leads, cares for, and protects us. If you look back over your life, you may be able to recognize some of the times when He has worked to get your attention and tell you He loves you.

What about the trials of life? Is God speaking to us through those? God's character can be seen in the midst of trying circumstances, and our faith and endurance is often developed when we look at trials through the lens of Calvary. God's love for you was proven at the cross: "For God so loved the world that He gave His only begotten Son" (John 3:16). He can never act toward you in a way other than love. Even His judgments and discipline are based on love. He is all-knowing and all-powerful; the decisions He makes for you are always best. God always leads His children as they would choose to be led if they could see the end from the beginning.

Many ask, *If God is so loving, why do so many bad things happen to good and innocent people?*

1. Because of our own choices. God does not force the will of anyone. He respects each person's right to choose whether or not they will obey Him and follow His will by doing as He directs. He lets us experience the results of our own choices.
2. Because of the choices of others. We all have an impact on each other's lives. The ill choices of Adam and Eve, our parents, civil leaders, drunk drivers, and others all affect our lives adversely. The innocent suffer from the wrong decisions of others.
3. Because of the violation of natural law. Objects fall, ice is slippery, and machinery fails. When the physical laws that govern our world are broken, accidents happen and people get hurt.
4. Because of the adversary. If you claim to be a Christian, Satan is allowed to test your loyalty and commitment to God. Those who have rejected God are at the dubious mercy of the evil one. Satan hates God. Since he can't hurt God directly, he causes God pain by hurting those God loves. He hurts those we care about to cause us pain as well.

When faced with a tragedy or hardship, many people have a hard time continuing to trust God because they know He could have stopped it and chose not to. God can keep bad things from happening to His children, and He does so more often than we realize. We must understand that because of the rules of the great controversy between God and Satan, the choices and circumstances that affect our lives may not be the best, but when we are surrendered to His loving care, He takes those less-than-perfect circumstances and choices and works them out for our ultimate benefit. He will always give us either strength to bear our trials or a way of escape. He promises that when we place ourselves in His hands, He will make all things come out for the best (Rom. 8:28).

Remember, God can see the big picture that we cannot. We are like children, incapable of understanding decisions for our future good that bring disappointment now. Rather than staring blindly at your hurts and dashed hopes, seek to understand God's perspective in each circumstance.

Talking to God

Some have said that prayer is like opening the heart to God as to a friend. Come to Him as you are, with your hopes, doubts, and questions. Share your concerns, your joys, and struggles. Persevere in learning of Him and talking to Him; you will come to experience His great and unfailing love; His power and wisdom; the kindness, beauty, and compassion of His character; and the joy of doing His will. You will learn to trust Him and know that He loves you and will never harm you.

Gratitude

Gratitude is a choice to be thankful and count your blessings rather than dwell on the troubles and hardships of your life. When you choose to be thankful for the good things in life, you will find yourself enjoying a happier frame of mind. Make a list every night of at least 10 things for which you are thankful. A little gratitude does wonders for all our relationships. Expressing your thanks to God will foster your trust and love for Him.

While there are many studies that show the health benefits of various positive mental attitudes, one of the most interesting pieces of evidence is the placebo effect. Placebos are commonly used to test new medicines. One test group is given the test drug, while the other is given a useless look-alike. Placebo subjects often report results as good as or better than those receiving the real medicine. Mental outlook has an extremely powerful influence on physical health. Attitude can make the difference in whether or not one recovers from a major illness. Grief, anxiety, discontent, remorse, guilt, distrust, anger, fear, and resentment cause stress and wear down the body, resulting in a weakened immune system and poor health. Courage, hope, faith, sympathy, love, contentment, forgiveness, joy, and gratitude promote health and prolong life. King Solomon said, "A merry heart doeth good like a medicine: but a broken spirit drieth the bones" (Proverbs 17:22).

Helping Others

The great law of life in the universe is a law of service. God provides for every living thing; Christ came to the earth to serve and give His life for mankind; the angels are occupied in caring for the needs of humanity.

The same law of service is seen throughout nature. The birds and animals; the trees, grass, and flowers; the sun, moon, and stars—all provide something of benefit to others.

Is the world a better place because you are here? Seek to live a life of service and benefit to others. Go out of your way to be kind to someone today. Whether that person is grateful or not, kindness is rewarding; giving is a condition of healthy living, a law of mental well-being.

Most of us find that when we're not in good health, it is easy to focus our attention on our needs and difficulties. Yet, getting our minds off ourselves and working for the good of others is often just what we need to give us the strength to get well. It also reminds us that we are not the only ones with problems; in fact, ours are smaller than the ones many people face.

YEARNING FOR REST

A vital part of a healthful lifestyle is getting the right quantity and quality of sleep. During this time the body grows, repairs damage, and restores energy, preparing itself for another day of activity. When the body is deprived of sleep, it is unable to rebuild and recharge itself. There is an increase in irritability; meanwhile, creativity, concentration, and efficiency suffer. Sleep deprivation impairs the brain, causing judgment and values to suffer. If sleep continues to be denied, exhaustion, depression, delusions, paranoia, and hallucinations can result. Losing as little as three hours of sleep in a single night can cut the effectiveness of your immune system in half. In a classic health study, it was found that people who regularly slept seven to eight hours each night had a lower death rate and lived longer than those who got more or less than that. The slowed reaction time and decreased concentration from lack of sleep led to a well-documented increase of accidents both fatal and nonfatal. Some estimates show that as many as 30 percent of fatal automobile accidents are caused by a driver falling asleep at the wheel.

In the U.S. fatigue is one of the most common reasons for visiting a physician. Many people have been sleepy for so long that they don't know what it is like to feel wide awake. Do you nod off whenever you're not active, need an alarm clock to wake up, or sleep longer on your days off? If so, you are probably not getting enough sleep.

Some ways to improve the quality of your sleep:

- Follow a regular exercise program in the fresh air and sunshine. The body will be more willing to rest if it has been active.

- Don't have a heavy evening meal. When the body has to finish the digestion process after you go to bed, you won't get the proper quality of rest.
- Have a regular sleeping schedule. Go to bed at the same time and get up at the same time, including weekends. It has been observed that the most efficient sleep occurs between 9 p.m. and midnight.
- Relax your body and mind. Take a warm bath; drink a cup of herbal tea, such as catnip or hops; enjoy some quiet reading or pleasant music; do something pleasant and soothing.
- Avoid stimulants like television, tobacco, nicotine, and caffeine.
- Avoid upsetting arguments, conversations, and confrontations in the evening. Before bedtime set your worries and anxieties aside. Ask forgiveness and make restitution to those you may have hurt; obtain a clear conscience.
- Refrain from alcohol; it interferes with the body's ability to rebuild while sleeping. Check your medications for side effects that interfere with sleep.
- A dark, cool, comfortable, tidy, quiet, sleeping area with an abundant supply of fresh air will soothe the body and encourage rest.
- Count the blessings, privileges, and benefits in your life.

Our bodies require more than just a daily period of sleep. At creation God provided for a weekly rest, the Sabbath. This is a whole day without work when the week's cares are set aside for quality time with God, our families, and other people. This rest is indispensable for total health—it's like an oasis in the midst of our busy lives, and it is very important for stress reduction. A longer period of recreation, a relaxing vacation, is also important from time to time to refresh and renew us. If we work continuously, we impose a strain upon our health and set ourselves up for disease.

How to schedule health into your day:

1. Rise early and drink two 8-ounce glasses of water.
2. Spend time seeking to know God through Bible study and prayer.
3. Do 15 minutes to an hour of exercise.
4. Eat a good breakfast.
5. During the morning, drink two or three 8-ounce glasses of water and avoid snacking.
6. Eat a moderate lunch followed by a stroll outside. Breathe deeply.
7. During the afternoon, drink two or three more glasses of water. No snacks.
8. Eat a very light evening meal or skip supper altogether and take a walk instead.
9. Change your pace in the evening; do something physical if your daytime work is mostly mental, or vice versa. Work in some family time. Drink at least one more glass of water.
10. Before you go to sleep, list 10 things for which you are thankful.
11. Go to bed in good time (one hour's rest before midnight is worth two after).

Chapter 5

Immune-Enhancing Foods and Supplements

The immune-enhancing supplements and foods found in this section are recommended for children and adults of all ages. These nutrients are essential and should be acquired as part of whole foods when possible. When this is not possible, specific nutrients may be supplemented in the diet. While generally regarded as safe and effective, these non-drug supplements should be used as directed on the labels or as recommended by a natural-remedies healthcare practitioner. Dosages will vary according to age and other factors, including past medical history, current nutritional status, and weight. Try to obtain vegetarian sources of supplements.

The following food nutrients help in increasing our immunity:

Vitamin A and Beta-Carotene

Sources: fruits and vegetables, especially the brightly colored ones.

Supplementation with vitamin A has been shown to reduce the severity of measles infections. Vitamin A deficiency increases susceptibility to any infection. For children and adults, the best vegetarian source is brightly colored fruits and vegetables. Seven to 11 servings of fruits and vegetables are recommended each day.

Beta-carotene has gained tremendous stature in the nutritional world. In recent years, researchers have discovered that beta-carotene not only functions as a precursor to vitamin A but also works on its own to maintain health. Beta-carotene is among the most powerful of anti-oxidant nutrients. As such, it can help guard against the development of cancer.

Beta-carotene is not toxic to the liver even in high doses. Large doses increase the body's demands for vitamin E. If you do take a large dose, such as 30 to 60 milligrams of beta-carotene (equivalent to 50,000 to 100,000 units of vitamin A activity), increase vitamin E to 1,000 to 2,000 units per day.[73]

Vitamin C

Sources: bell pepper, broccoli, Brussels sprouts, cauliflower, fruit juices, lemon juice, mustard greens, oranges, papaya, strawberries, and kiwi fruit.

Foods with vitamin C increase the production of infection-fighting white blood cells and increase levels of interferon, the antibody that coats cell surfaces to prevent the entry of viruses.

Vitamin E

Sources: almonds, broccoli, chard, mustard greens, olives, papaya, sunflower seeds, and turnip greens.

Vitamin E stimulates the production of natural "killer" cells (cells that seek out and destroy germs and cancer cells). Vitamin E enhances the production of B-cells, the immune cells that produce antibodies that destroy bacteria. Vitamin E may also reverse some of the decline in immune response commonly seen in aging.

Vitamin B Complex

The vitamin B complex consists of eight water-soluble vitamins. The B vitamins work together to boost metabolism, enhance the immune system and nervous system, keep the skin and muscles healthy, encourage cell growth and division, and bring other benefits to your body. Brewer's yeast and whole grains are the best sources of the B vitamins .

Thiamine (B1)

Sources: asparagus, leafy greens, vegetables, cereals, sunflower seeds, legumes, berries, and wheat germ.

Vitamin B1 serves as a catalyst in carbohydrate metabolism and helps synthesize nerve-regulating substances. Deficiency can cause heart swelling, leg cramps, and muscular weakness. The Recommended Dietary Allowance (RDA) is 1.5 mg.

Riboflavin (B2)

Sources: asparagus, cereals, cranberries, mushrooms, romaine lettuce, pasta, and bread.

Vitamin B2 helps metabolize fats, carbohydrates, and respiratory proteins. A deficiency can result in skin lesions and light sensitivity. The vitamin is good for the skin, nails, eyes, mouth, lips, and tongue, and it is believed to help protect against cancer. The RDA is 1.3 mg for adults.

Niacin (B3)

Sources: asparagus, cranberries, mushrooms, tomatoes, nuts, dried beans, and peas.

Vitamin B3—also known as vitamin P, or vitamin PP—helps release energy from nutrients. It can reduce cholesterol and prevent and treat arteriosclerosis, among other benefits. Too little B3 can result in pellagra, a disease with symptoms that include sunburn, diarrhea, irritability, swollen tongue, and mental confusion. Too much B3 can result in liver damage. The RDA is 14-18 mg per day for adults.

Pantothenic acid (B5)

Sources: whole grain cereals, legumes; it may be found in some quantity in nearly every food.

Vitamin B5 has a role in the metabolism of fats, carbohydrates, and proteins. Deficiency can result in fatigue, allergies, nausea, and abdominal pain. The RDA is 10 mg.

Pyridoxine (B6)

Sources: bell peppers, cauliflower, cranberries, mustard greens, turnips, spinach, green beans, avocados, whole grains, bread, and bananas.

Vitamin B6 helps the body to absorb and metabolize amino acids, to use fats, and to form red blood cells. Deficiency in the vitamin may result in smooth tongue, skin disorders, dizziness, nausea, anemia, convulsions, and kidney stones. The RDA ranges from 1.3 to 2 mg depending on age and gender.

Biotin (B7)

Sources: beans, bread, brewer's yeast, cauliflower, legumes, molasses, nuts, oatmeal, wheat germ and whole grains, soy, mushrooms, and bananas.

Vitamin B7 or vitamin H helps form fatty acids and assists in the release of energy from carbohydrates. There have been no known cases of deficiency among humans. The RDA is 30 micrograms.

Folic acid (B9)

Sources: asparagus, beets, broccoli, lentils, parsley, romaine lettuce, spinach, turnip greens and other green leafy vegetables, and nuts.

Vitamin B9, folic acid or folate, also goes by the name of vitamin M or vitamin B-c. Folic acid enables the body to form hemoglobin. It helps treat anemia and sprue. Deficiency is rare, although folic acid is particularly important in pregnancy. Consuming adequate folic acid before and during pregnancy helps prevent neural tube defects in newborns, including spina bifida. The RDA for both men and women is 400 micrograms, but women who are pregnant or planning to become pregnant should consume 600 micrograms a day. When breastfeeding, the recommendation is 500 micrograms.

Cobalamin or Cyanocobalamin (B12)

Sources: fortified breakfast cereal, soy milk, yeast extracts, and wheat germ.

Vitamin B12 is central to immune processes because, without adequate B12, white blood cells can't mature and multiply. It also assists the function of the nervous system and the formation of red blood cells. If the body is unable to absorb sufficient B12, pernicious anemia can result. Therefore, vegetarians are encouraged to check and supplement if necessary. The RDA for adult males and females is 2.4 micrograms.

Zinc

Sources: mushrooms and legumes.

This valuable mineral increases the production and effectiveness of white blood cells that fight infection. Zinc also increases killer cells that fight against cancer, and it helps white cells release more antibodies. Zinc also increases the number of infection-fighting T-cells, especially in elderly people, who are often deficient in zinc and whose immune systems often weaken with age. The anti-infection hype around zinc is controversial. While some studies claim that zinc supplements in the form of lozenges can lower the incidence and severity of infections, other studies have failed to show this correlation. A word of caution: too much zinc (more than 75 milligrams a day) in the form of supplements can inhibit immune function.

Chromium

Sources: brewer's yeast, onions, whole grains, bran cereals, tomatoes, and potatoes.

Many people do not get enough chromium in their diet due to food processing methods that remove the naturally occurring chromium in commonly consumed foods. Recent research in animal models shows that chromium can enhance the ability of white blood cells to respond to infection.

Selenium

Sources: Brazil nuts, brown rice, soy cheese, garlic, mushrooms, sunflower seeds, and whole grains.

This mineral increases natural killer cells and mobilizes cancer-fighting cells.

Probiotics

Supplementation with probiotic products provides another unique type of protection against most common infections, allergies, and cancers. *Probiotics* is the name given to the "friendly" bacteria that maintain a healthy intestinal flora, an essential aspect of overall health.

Probiotics prevent the overgrowth of undesirable intestinal bacteria and microorganisms that produce putrefactive and carcinogenic toxins. If harmful bacteria dominate the intestines, essential vitamins and enzymes are not produced, and the level of harmful substances rises, leading to cancer, liver and kidney disease, hypertension, and arteriosclerosis.

Well-known probiotics include *Lactobacillus acidophilus* and *Bifidobacterium bifidum*. Another probiotic that has recently generated a great deal of interest is the friendly yeast known as *Saccharomyces boulardii*, an organism that belongs to the brewer's yeast family. It is not a permanent resident of the intestine, but taken orally it produces lactic acid and some B vitamins and has an overall immune-enhancing effect.

Probiotics are considered to be very safe and well tolerated in the usual dosages prescribed. Highly sensitive individuals have reported the occasional occurrence of indigestion (nausea, heartburn) that disappeared when the supplement was discontinued or the brand of probiotic was changed.

Vaccinations, x-rays, prescription antibiotics, steroids, chlorine, tobacco, caffeine, alcohol, and sugar inhibit probiotics. There is also some evidence that casein, a milk protein found in most commercial dairy products, inhibits probiotic growth. The antibiotics found in dairy products are also a factor in suppressing probiotics. A diet high in complex carbohydrates (vegetables, fruits, whole grains, legumes) encourages the proliferation of most probiotics.

Nondigestible food factors that selectively stimulate the growth and activity of probiotics in the gut are referred to as "prebiotics." The best example of a prebiotic is FOS (fructo-oligo-saccharides).This substance is found naturally in many vegetables, grains, and fruits, including Jerusalem artichokes, chicory, burdock, garlic, and onions. In Japan, FOS is widely used as a sweetener.

Probiotic sources include cultured/fermented soy products like soymilk, tofu, tempeh, and miso. Other, lesser-known food sources of probiobtics are sauerkraut and sourdough breads. If dietary sources are not easily available, supplemental probiotic powders and capsules are good alternatives.

Larch arabinogalactan

Larch arabinogalactan is found in a wide range of plants, including carrots, radishes, black beans, pears, wheat, and tomatoes, but most abundantly in the larch tree. Immune-enhancing herbs like echinacea also contain significant amounts.

Larch arabinogalactan has potent immune-enhancing properties and is an excellent source of dietary fiber. Supplementation will lower the generation and subsequent absorption of ammonia, a potent neurotoxin. It also protects colon cells against cancer-promoting agents.

Immune-Modulating Botanicals

Using a combination of herbs, minerals, vitamins, and other foods increases interferon and T-cell production and can further bolster immunity. A substance called interferon is produced naturally by the body's white cells to fight off and prevent viral and other infections. A fever stimulates the body to make more interferon. This is one of the reasons why natural-remedies practitioners are against the use of drugs to suppress fevers. Interferon can stimulate the immune system to produce more of the disease-fighting T-cells.

Many natural substances have been shown to stimulate the body's production of interferon. Some of the best known and documented ones are listed below:

Astragalus: This Chinese herb enhances antibody reaction to antigens, increases T-lymphocyte activity, improves symptoms of many HIV-related problems, and increases the body's production of interferon. In traditional Chinese medicine, astragalus enjoys a long history of use as an immune system booster and potent tonic for increasing energy levels. Astragalus has been proven to enhance immunity in cancer patients and offsets bone marrow suppression and gastrointestinal toxicity caused by chemotherapy and radiation. No side effects have been reported.

Boneset: Native American Indians use this herb successfully for the treatment of colds, flu, coughs, fevers, indigestion, and pain. It has antiseptic properties, promotes sweating, is antiviral, and boosts the immune system by enhancing the body's own secretion of interferon.

Echinacea (*Echinacea angustifolia*): North American Indians have used echinacea as a treatment for toothaches, snake bites, insect bites or stings, and all types of infections. It has a reputation as a blood purifier and also has interferon-like properties. It fights both strep and staph infections, candida (yeast infections), and can kill fungi. It has been used successfully for blood poisoning, ulcers, tuberculosis, childhood infections of every kind, and a long list of skin, digestive, and immune system disorders.

Germanium: Many practitioners use this trace mineral for the treatment of chronic fatigue, allergies, infections, and cancer. A good source of naturally occurring germanium is Korean ginseng.

Licorice: Many of the world's cultures have used licorice as a tonic and energy booster, as well as for the treatment of infections and female disorders. Licorice has anti-inflammatory and antiallergic properties. The two licorice components, glycyrrhizm and glycyrrhetinic acid, stimulate the production of interferon by the body. Licorice is very helpful for coughs, colds, and flu, and heals inflamed mucous membranes in the respiratory tract.

Medicinal Mushrooms: Reishi, Maitake, Shiitake, and Kombucha, among others, stimulate many aspects of the immune system, including the production of interferon.

Oil of Oregano (*Origanum vulgare*): This oil is well known in the Mediterranean world for its ability to slow down food spoilage through its antibacterial, antiviral, antifungal, antiparasitic, and antioxidant activity. Oregano oil boosts the immune system. It also acts as a free radical scavenger, protecting against toxins and preventing further tissue damage while encouraging healing.

Pau d'Arco: This herb is well known for its antifungal properties and its stimulating effect on the immune system. Several anecdotal reports have indicated that it could help fight cancer.

Vitamin A and Beta-carotene: Both nutrients boost interferon production.

Vitamin C and Bioflavonoids: Vitamins C boosts interferon production. Especially beneficial are pycnogenols like grape seed extract, pine bark extract, and bilberry, as well as quercetin, hesperidin, and catechin.

Wheat Grass: This "superfood" is rich in vitamins, minerals, amino acids, and enzymes. It also enhances interferon production. It is taken in juice form.

Chapter 6

Botanical Medicine

How to Understand and Use Healing Herbs

Herbal medicine is part of our traditional and ancient wisdom. We are very fortunate that this wisdom has not been totally lost following the introduction of synthetic drug therapy.

Many of our modern drugs are synthesized by basing the chemistry on a particular component of plant medicine. Scientists are realizing, however, that individual constituents of a plant do not have the same effect as the whole plant. First, a single plant contains an enormous number of constituents, only some of which have been analyzed. Several components probably work together synergistically to achieve a given effect. This is why many herbs are actually more effective in the long run than drug treatments, which tend to give dramatic but short-lived benefits. *Herbs are not drugs.*

In this section I will emphasize botanical medicine as a method for prevention and treatment of disease and as an alternative to vaccines. Current scientific research around the world is confirming the beneficial constituents and actions of herbal remedies. Natural-remedies practitioners have long found these actions both relevant and useful in preventing disease.

This chapter also provides specific instructions for preparing and using medicinal herbs. You will need this information in order to use the next chapter.

Adaptogen: An adaptogen produces an increase in bodily resistance and vitality, helping the body adapt to and defend against the effects of environmental stress factors. Adaptogens work in three ways: (A) They show a nonspecific activity by increasing the body's ability to resist physical, chemical, or biological noxious agents. (B) They have a normalizing influence independent of the pathological state. (C) They are innocuous and do not influence normal body functions more than required.

Alteratives: This term designates a class of agents which alter the course of morbid conditions. Alteratives work by (A) modifying the nutritive processes while promoting waste, (B) stimulating secretion and adsorption, and (C) eliminating morbid deposits.

Medicinal Actions of Herbs

The adaptogenic and alterative actions are well suited for body systems. A single herbal agent may have primary, secondary, tertiary, or other actions. Following is a list of medicinal actions and herbal examples:

Adaptogen
Herbs that normalize and restore body functions and increase the body's nonspecific resistance to stress: ginseng, licorice, nettle, and astragalus.

Alterative
Also known as blood purifiers. Herbs that gradually restore health and vitality to the body: burdock, red clover, nettle, Oregon grape, alfalfa, gota kola, marshmallow, dong quai, and ginseng.

Analgesic/Anodyne
Substances that relieve pain: scullcap, valerian, passion flower, catnip, and chamomile.

Antacid
Substances that neutralize excess acid in the stomach and intestinal tract: dandelion, fennel, slippery elm, catnip, mullein, and meadowsweet.

Anthelmintic
Herbs that expel or kill worms: garlic, onion, wormwood, rue, and thyme.

Antibiotic or Antimicrobial
Substances that inhibit the growth of or destroy bacteria, viruses, or amoebas: echinacea, goldenseal, myrrh, chaparral, juniper berries, thyme, and garlic.

Anticatarrhal
Substances that eliminate or counteract the formation of mucus: cayenne, ginger, sage, cinnamon, anise, gota kola, mullein, comfrey, and wild cherry bark.

Anti-inflammatory
Herbs that reduce inflammation: St. John's wort, calendula, arnica, licorice, chamomile, and wild yam.

Antilithic
Herbs that prevent or dissolve and discharge urinary and biliary stones and gravel: dandelion, cleavers, corn silk, and uva ursi. For gallbladder: Oregon grape and chaparral.

Antiphlogistic
Reduces localized inflammations, itching, and swelling.

Antipyretic
Cooling herbs used to reduce fevers: alfalfa, basil, gota kola, skullcap, chickweed, and yarrow.

Antiseptic
Substances that can be applied to the skin to prevent the growth of bacteria: goldenseal, calendula, chaparral, myrrh, and the oils of thyme, garlic, pine, juniper berries, and sage.

Antispasmodic
Herbs that prevent or relax muscle spasms: lobelia, dong quai, black and blue cohosh, scullcap, valerian, kava kava, raspberry leaves, and rue.

Aphrodisiac
Substances used to improve sexual potency and power: damiana, saw palmetto, ginseng, sarsaparilla, kava kava, and burdock.

Aromatic
A pleasant-smelling and tasting herb that stimulates the gastrointestinal system and improves the taste of medicines and foods: lavender, peppermint, angelica, cinnamon, dill, and citrus peel.

Astringent
Herb causing constriction of tissues: witch hazel, white oak bark, yellow dock, uva ursi, calendula, myrrh, horsetail, and blackberry root.

Bitter
Herb that stimulates gastric function: hops, mugwort, and dandelion.

Carminative
Promotes digestion, expels gas, and relieves gripping: anise, fennel, chamomile, peppermint, caraway, and ginger.

Cholagogue
Herbs taken to promote the flow and discharge of bile into the small intestine: goldenseal, Oregon grape, dandelion, and wild yam.

Demulcent
Soothing substances taken internally that protect and sooth the digestive tract. They trigger reflex mechanisms that travel through the spinal nerves, effectively reducing inflammation and irritation in the respiratory and urinary systems: comfrey, marshmallow, slippery elm, and corn silk.

Diaphoretic
Substances that promote perspiration: elder, yarrow, osha, and ginger.

Diuretic
Substances that increase the flow of urine: dandelion, couch grass, uva ursi, plantain, and horsetail.

Emetic
Substances that induce vomiting and cause the stomach to empty: lobelia, ipecac, elecampane, and blessed thistle.

Emmenagogue
Herbs that promote menstruation: pennyroyal, juniper berries, myrrh, black cohosh, rue, and wild ginger.

Emollients
Substances that sooth and soften the skin: marshmallow, comfrey root, slippery elm, chickweed, and plantain.

Expectorant
Herbs that help expel mucus from the lungs and throat. Herbs that stimulate the nerves and muscles of the respiratory system to manifest a cough. An example is elecampane.

Relaxing expectorant
Herbs that reduce tension in lung tissue, often easing tightness, allowing natural coughing and flow of mucus to occur: coltsfoot, licorice, and hyssop.

Amphoteric expectorant

Herbs that stimulate or relax the respiratory systems, using the body's choice, which is necessary: lobelia, mullein, horehound, elder, and garlic.

Febrifuge

Herbs that assist the body in reducing fevers: catnip, elder, and peppermint.

Galactogogue

Substance that increase the secretion of milk: anise, blessed thistle, fennel, and vervain.

Hemostatic

Herbs that are internal astringents that arrest internal hemorrhaging: blackberry, cayenne, cranesbill, mullein, goldenseal, horsetail, uva ursi, yellow dock, witch hazel, and shepherd's purse.

Hepatic

Herbs that strengthen and tone the liver: Oregon grape, agrimony, dandelion, goldenseal, wild yam.

Hypnotic

Herbs that have a powerful relaxant and sedative action and help induce sleep: hops, valerian, and wild lettuce.

Hypotensive

Herbs that reduce elevated blood pressure: crampbark, garlic, onion, yarrow, and hawthorn berries.

Laxative

Substances that stimulate bowel movement: cascara sagrada, yellow dock, and rhubarb root.

Lymphatic

Herbs that support the health and activity of the lymphatic system: cleaver, calendula, and echinacea.

Nervine

Herbs that calm nervous tension and nourish the nerves: chamomile, hops, oats, scullcap, and St. John's wort.

Oxytocic
Substances that stimulate uterine contractions to assist and induce labor: black and blue cohosh, rue, squawvine, and uva ursi.

Pectoral
Herbs that generally strengthen and heal the respiratory system: elecampane, coltsfoot, comfrey, and mullein.

Rubefacient
Substances that increase the flow of blood to the surface of the skin and produce redness. They draw inflammation and congestions from deeper areas: nettle, mustard seed, cayenne, horseradish, pine, and thyme oil.

Sedative
Herbs that quiet the nervous system: valerian, scullcap, passion flower, wood betony, chamomile, and catnip.

Sialogogue
Herbs that promote the secretion and flow of saliva: echinacea, cayenne, ginger, and licorice.

Stimulants
Herbs that increase the energy of the body, quicken circulation, break up obstructions and congestion: cayenne, ginger, horseradish, and wormwood.

Styptic
Herbs that arrest or reduce external bleeding due to astringent action on blood vessels: yarrow, horsetail, cayenne, and plantain.

Tonic
Herbs that stimulate nutrition by improving the assimilation of essential nutrients by the organs; they improve systemic tone, giving increased vigor, energy, and strength to the tissues of either specific organs or to the whole body. Most tonics have an affinity for a particular system. Nerve tonics: skullcap, lobelia, valerian, and oats. Heart tonics: hawthorn, ginseng, and motherwort. Stomach tonics: agrimony, elecampane, and gentian. Liver tonics: dandelion, sassafras, and cascara. Biliary tonics: Oregon grape, goldenseal, rhubarb, parsley, and wild yam. Sexual tonics: damiana, ginseng, dong quai, burdock, and licorice.

Vasodilator
Herbs that expand blood vessels and allow increased circulation: gingko, feverfew, Siberian ginseng, ginger, and cayenne.

Vulnerary
Herbs that help the body to heal wounds by promoting cell growth and repair: comfrey, calendula, chickweed, St. John's wort, marshmallow, aloe vera, rosemary, thyme, and slippery elm.

Antimicrobials

What is an Antimicrobial?
The antimicrobial herbs can help the body to destroy or resist pathogenic microorganisms. With herbal remedies it is possible to help the body strengthen its own resistance to infective organisms and throw off the illness. While some plant remedies contain chemicals which are strongly antiseptic or constitute a specific poison to certain organisms, in general we are talking about plants that aid the natural immune processes.

Many of the plants that have this action are also anti-inflammatory, antiviral, antiparasitic, and so on. The body can benefit from supportive and preventative help that bypasses the need for chemical intervention in an emergency.

How Antimicrobials Work
Some research work has been done on these antimicrobial remedies, and in such cases an active ingredient has occasionally been found. An example is the German research into the excellent remedy echinacea, where a chemical with antibacterial properties was discovered. It is called echinacein. The plant also contains a volatile oil that is anti-staphylococcal, an amide of the echinacein that is insecticidal, others that are antifungal, and a polypeptide that attacks bacteria. Echinacea also has action against viruses, apparently by inhibiting an enzyme used by viruses to break down cell walls.

Herbs rich in volatile oils are often directly effective by killing microorganisms. Examples of these herbs would be garlic, thyme, and eucalyptus. Another way in which herbs can work to remove infection is by direct or indirect stimulation of the body's own immune system. Myrrh is an example of this.

Each system of the body has plants that are particularly suited to it, some of which are antimicrobial. (Consult a general textbook of herbal medicine to learn more about herbal actions and which antimicrobial remedies may be best suited for each system of the body.) By the nature of infection and the body's immune response to it, a general systemic treatment is always appropriate, even if done in conjunction with specific local remedies. The following antimicrobial herbal agents may be used both locally and generally:

Antimicrobial Herbal Agents

Aloe	Buchu
Echinacea	Tea tree
Goldenseal	Elderberry
Garlic	Peppermint
Grapefruit	Lemon balm
Olive leaf	Thyme
Calendula	Sage
Myrrh	Rosemary
Chinese skullcap	Lomatium root
Japanese honeysuckle	Osha root
Lemon juice	Vinegar

How to Prepare Herbal Remedies

Standard Tea Mixture for Adults:
(one cup)
1. Place one teaspoon of dried herbs (one-half teaspoon of powdered herbs) or one tablespoon of fresh green herbs in a cup and pour boiling water onto herbs. Cover and steep for 20 minutes.
2. Strain liquid into an empty cup.
3. Drink as advised in treatment section.

(one quart)
1. Place equal amounts of three different types of the dried herbs in a large plastic zipper bag and shake well. Double the amount is required for fresh herbs.
2. Place three tablespoons (dried) or six tablespoons (fresh) of this herb mixture in a teapot and pour boiling water onto herbs. Cover and steep for 20 minutes.
3. Strain liquid into an empty quart jar and add additional water to make one quart.
4. Drink as advised in treatment section.

Infusion:

An infusion is made like a tea. Use this method for the softer, green, or flowering parts of the plant. Place the herbs or herb mixture in a pot. Pour boiling water onto mixture and leave to steep for 10 minutes before straining. A general guide is to use one teaspoon of dried herbs per cup of water or one tablespoon of fresh herbs per cup of water. Quantities may vary according to the freshness and quality of the herb used and the strength of the infusion required.

Decoctions:

Use this method for the harder, woodier root, bark, berries, or seeds of the plant. Using a similar quantity as for an infusion, place the plant material in a saucepan, pour on the water, cover the pot, bring to a boil, and simmer for 10 to 15 minutes before straining. If steam escapes, add a little more water.

Tinctures:

A tincture is an extraction of the herb using water or alcohol. Put 4 ounces of finely chopped or ground dried herb into a container that can be tightly closed. (If the herb is fresh, use twice the amount.) Pour one pint of 30-percent grain alcohol or 60-proof vodka on the herbs and close the container tightly.

Keep the container in a warm place for two weeks and shake well twice daily. Then decant the liquid into a bowl. Pour the finished tincture into a dark-colored, tightly capped bottle. A standard dose is 5 ml of tincture in a glass of water three times a day.

Glycerites:

A glycerite is a preparation that uses glycerin to extract the constituents from an herb. Glycerin is both a solvent and a preservative and good for preparing children's remedies because of its sweet taste and lack of alcohol. Such preparations can be stirred into juice. They are also a good choice for people who do not want the alcohol in tinctures. Since glycerin can be chemically synthesized, it is best to ask for pure vegetable glycerin when purchasing.

Herbal glycerites may be prepared using two methods. In one method, dried or fresh herbs are blended with pure vegetable glycerin. The resulting mixture is shaken each day for two weeks, then pressed or squeezed through a filter to produce a clear product. Alternatively, a glycerite may be prepared by slowly evaporating the alcohol from a tincture and then adding a volume of glycerin equal to the original amount of alcohol.

Capsules:

The capsule is another convenient way of using herbs. They are often available in plastic or glass bottles. Some individuals prefer filling their own capsules. Capsules may contain any part of the plant: leaf, stalk, flower, or root, all ground to a fine powder. A standard dose is one to three capsules three times a day.

Tablets:

I believe it is best to purchase herbal tablets rather than attempting to prepare them. It is a laborious undertaking and not exact.

For Slippery Elm Preparations:

This is a common remedy with its own set of procedures. Following are brief instructions and dosage information:

- Decoction: Prepare by simmering for an hour or longer one part powdered bark to 8 parts water. This will make a mucilaginous drink that can be taken as often as needed. May also be added to juice or oatmeal.
- Infusion: Prepare by pouring 2 cups boiling water over 4 grams (roughly 2 tablespoons) of powdered bark and then steeping for 3 to 5 minutes. Drink three times per day.
- Capsules: Take two capsules (250 to 500 mg) three times daily.
- Lozenges: Follow dosing instructions on label.
- External application: Mix coarse powdered bark with boiling water to make a poultice.

Dosages

Herbal remedies are usually taken three times a day, whatever the form of preparation. In a very acute situation, such as influenza, you may wish to take the remedy more frequently.

When treating an acute illness, take the herbs for several days until the symptoms pass. For symptoms that persist following an illness, most herbs may be taken safely for up to six weeks. If any symptoms remain after that time or if conditions become more acute, you should consult a natural-remedies healthcare practitioner or other healthcare specialist.

Standard Adult Dose: one to three capsules taken three times a day.

Standard Adult Tea Dose: one cup taken three to four times a day.

Doses for Babies and Children

Doses given in previous instructions are for normal adults. Doses for babies and children should be reduced in proportion with body weight. The following table shows doses for babies and children expressed as a percentage of the adult dose.

Age	Avg. weight (lbs) for age	Percentage of Adult Dose
Birth	4 – 8 lbs	5%
6 months	17 lbs	10%
1 year	21 lbs	15%
2 years	28 lbs	20%
4	40 lbs	25%
6	48 lbs	30%
7	56 lbs	35%
8	62 lbs	40%
9	68 lbs	45%
10	77 lbs	50%
11	84 lbs	55%
12	100 lbs	60%
13	110 lbs	70%
14	127 lbs	80%
15	136 lbs	90%
16 and over	142 + lbs	100%

Only gentle herbs should be used with babies and young children.

While babies are being breastfed, herbs should generally be taken by the mother, so the baby may obtain them through the breast milk. The mother should take the adult dose.

Children may not like herbs that do not taste nice. Herbs may be added to foods or drinks to improve taste.

Interpolation may be used with the above table. For example, if a 4-year-old uses 25 percent of the adult dose, and a 6-year-old uses 30 percent of the adult dose, a 5-year-old may use 27.5 percent of the adult dose. Alternatively, the dose of the nearest younger age is close enough. For example, the dose of a 4-year-old (25 percent), is close enough for a 5-year-old.

Do not take any herbs in therapeutic dose during pregnancy without first consulting a natural-remedies practitioner or other healthcare specialist.

A Plan of Action

There *are* alternatives to conventional medical immunizations. If you have chosen to opt out of conventional vaccines for yourself or your child, the next step is to develop a plan of action.

An in-depth and detailed knowledge of the various actions of herbal agents is not required to use this guide. However, if you desire to delve more deeply into medical plants and their uses, refer to the textbooks by David Hoffman and James Duke listed in the Appendix.

Use this book as a guideline and consult with a natural-remedies healthcare practitioner or other healthcare providers who support your decision and will work with you to minimize susceptibility to disease—the natural way. The next chapter will provide vital information to help you avoid using drugs, chemicals, and other harmful additives in your body. Read on!

Part II

Diseases and Alternatives to Vaccines

Chapter 7

How to Prevent and Treat Common Diseases

How to Use This Section

What follows is the heart of this book: a brief guide to natural remedies for common illnesses. When using these treatment plans, refer to Chapter 6 for instructions on how to prepare herbal remedies, for guidance in calculating doses, and for information about antimicrobials and the medicinal actions of herbs. For instructions on hydrotherapy (water treatment) procedures, refer to the Appendix (Notes on Hydrotherapy). Any deviations from the standard mixtures or measurements will be specified in the appropriate sections below.

The points below are highlighted because they occur so often in this chapter. They are emphasized to eliminate repetition.

- For all illnesses, apply **Optimum (IMMUNITY) Principles** (Chapter 4).
- Use **antimicrobial herbal agents** to prevent and treat diseases (Chapter 6).
- **Dosing information for adults and children** is located in Chapter 6.

CHOLERA

Cholera *(Vibrio cholera)* is an acute toxigenic disease of the gastrointestinal tract that tends to occur in epidemics. This organism grows in the small intestine and produces a toxin that causes severe diarrhea. It is spread by fecal-contaminated food and water, shellfish, and by flies. In the developed world cholera has disappeared due to improved sanitation and hygiene. The incubation period is two to seven days. Symptoms develop rapidly and can become dangerous in six to 12 hours. The symptoms include nausea, vomiting, abdominal cramps, and severe watery diarrhea ("rice-water" stools). Children become restless and go into stupor or have convulsions. The diarrhea causes dehydration and a fall in blood pressure, and fatalities are most often from circulatory failure.

The cholera vaccine is notoriously ineffective and not highly recommended because of the brief and incomplete immunity it confers.

HERBALS AND BOTANICALS: Agrimony (*Agrimonia eupatoria*), **Catnip** (*Nepeta cataria*), **Bayberry** (*Myrica cerifera*), **Blackberry Leaves** (*Rubus fruticosus*), **Black Cohosh** (*Cimicifuga racemosa*), **Boneset** (*Cimicifuga racemosa*), **Cranesbill** (*Geranium maculatum*), **Garlic** (*Allium sativum*), **Gentian** (*Gentiana lutea*), **Ginger** (*Zingiber officinale*), **Goldenseal** (*Hydrastis canadensis*), **Guava Leaves** (*Psidium guajava*), **Lemongrass** (*Cymbopogon citratus* syn. *Andropogon citrates*), **Lobelia** (*Lobelia inflata*), **Loosestrife** (*Lythrum Salicaria*), **Oak Bark** (*Quercus robar*), **Peppermint** (*Mentha x piperita*), **Marshmallow** (*Althaea officinalis*), **Myrrh** (*Commiphora myrrha*), **Stinging Nettle** (*Uritica dioical*), **Peach Leaf** (*Prunus persica*), **Pennyroyal** (*Mentha pulegium*), **Raspberry Leaf** (*Rubus idaeus*), **Ragwort** (*Senecio jacobaea*), **Red Clover** (*Trifolium pretense*), **Skunk Cabbage** (*Symplocarps foetidus*), **Slippery Elm** (*Ulmus fulva*), **Snakeroot** (*Polygala senega*), **Spearmint** (*Mentha spicata*)

FORM: Capsules, teas, and tablets

HERBAL PROPHYLAXIS AND TREATMENT:

Prevention: Avoid the consumption of contaminated food or water; wash hands. Use **antimicrobial herbs:** Take one capsule three times a day, three times a week (every other day) or one cup of tea made from any three-herb mixture, three times a week (every other day) for one to two weeks prior to traveling in an endemic cholera area or during an outbreak.

Treatment: Drink copious amounts of various fluids daily for their rehydration effect throughout the course of the illness and convalescence. Use **antitoxin herbs (goldenseal, gentian, bayberry, lemongrass)** and **antimicrobial herbs:** Take two to three capsules three times a day or one cup of tea made from any three-herb mixture three times a day for one week, then rotate combination of herbs each week until symptoms are gone.

- Cholera usually begins with watery diarrhea, which can be checked at once by the use of a high enema, as hot as tolerated, with **bayberry bark, white willow bark, wild cherry bark, catnip,** followed by antispasmodic teas: **peppermint, bayberry, catnip, raspberry leaves, peach leaves, sunflower leaves.** These combinations can be warm and soothing.
- Treatment should be directed mainly at replacing all of the liquids and important chemical elements/electrolytes lost from the bowels because of diarrhea.

- While diarrhea is in an active stage, patient should be kept warm, quiet, and in bed. An antispasmodic tea can be given with good benefit. **Skullcap, lobelia, myrrh, black cohosh,** and **skunk cabbage** may be given for bowel cramps. **Slippery elm** and **mullein tea** is nutritional and cleansing and can be given for the mucilaginous effect.
- **Lemongrass** may also be used to treat cholera because of its calming effect on the stomach.
- For vomiting give large amounts of **ragwort, boneset, pennyroyal, snakeroot**; after emetic action give small amounts of **peppermint, spearmint,** and **catnip** to sooth and settle the stomach.
- A **peppermint** enema is excellent for cholera, colon problems, and for convulsions and spasms in children.
- To strengthen the stomach and neutralize toxins use **goldenseal, gentian, bayberry.**
- For cholera fevers use **purple loosestrife** and **ginger.**
- The antimicrobial herbal agents may be used throughout the course of the disease.
- Hot fomentation (see hydrotherapy section in Appendix) over the bowel and the full length of the spine area for 15 to 20 minutes followed by a cold sponging is beneficial; repeat the alternating hot and cold for four repetitions. This may be done every three to four hours on a daily basis for severe cases. Finish the treatment with a shower or sponge bath.
- Linen and personal clothing should be laundered separately.
- Articles touched by patient should be disinfected.
- The best nutrition during cholera: oatmeal water, slippery elm water, and soy milk, progressing to a nutritious broth and then to a complete vegan diet.

CONTRAINDICATIONS: None

DIPHTHERIA

Diphtheria (*Corynebacterium diphtheriae*) is an infectious disease that typically strikes the upper respiratory tract, including the throat. This bacteria infection has a short incubation period (two to four days) and becomes very contagious. Due to improved hygiene, it is now rare in developed countries but is still significant in the developing world. Children are mostly affected, although during epidemics it may also be seen in adults. Many adults are naturally immune, and immunity can be established by a skin test. Immunization against diphtheria is part of the DTaP vaccine given routinely to infants.

Symptoms start with a sore throat, and the tonsils and larynx or sometimes the nose may become affected as the toxin builds up. The tonsils become covered with a grayish-white to yellow membrane that may extend over the soft palate and cannot be wiped off with a swab. In severe cases the membrane may obstruct the larynx, and breathing becomes obstructed and progresses to pneumonia. A generalized toxemia may also develop, causing a fall in blood pressure or paralysis. Any suspicion of paralysis should be referred to a doctor urgently, as this can also affect the ability to breathe. Reports as to the efficacy of the immunization vary greatly. Serious side effects, including death from anaphylactic shock, are well documented.

HERBALS AND BOTANICALS: Agrimony *(Agrimonia eupatoria)*, **Anise Seed** *(Pimpinella anisum)*, **Bayberry** *(Myrica cerifera)*, **Black Cohosh** *(Cimicifuga racemosa)*, **Bloodroot** *(Sanguinaria Canadensis)*, **Catnip** *(Nepeta cataria)*, **Cayenne** *(Capsicum annuum)*, **Chamomile** *(Matricaria recutita)*, **Chickweed** *(Stellaria Media)*, **Crampbark** *(Vifurnum opulus)*, **Echinacea Root** *(Echinacea purpurea)*, **Eucalyptus** *(Euacalyptys spp.)*, **Fennel** *(Foeniculum valgare)*, **Garlic** *(Alluum sativum)*, **Ginger** *(Zingiber officinale)*, **Goldenseal** *(Hydrastis Canadensis)*, **Lemon Juice** *(Citrus limonum)*, **Licorice** *(Glycyrrhiza glabra)*, **Lobelia** *(Lobelia inflata)*, **Mullein** *(Verbascum thapsus)*, **Myrrh** *(Commiphora molmol, C. myrrha)*, **Papaya** *(Carica papaya)*, **Peppermint** *(Mentha x piperita)*, **Persimmon Bark** *(Diospyros virginiana)*, **Ragwort** *(Senecio jacobaea)*, **Raspberry Leaves** *(Rubus idaeus)*, **Scotch Broom** *(Cytisus scoparius)*, **Skullcap** *(Scutellaria lateriflora)*, **Shepherd's Purse** *(Capsella bursa-pastoris)*, **Strawberry Leaves** *(Fragaria vesca)*, **Sumac Berry** *(Rhus glabra)*, **White Oak Bark** *(Quercus alba)*, **Wild Alum Root** *(Pelargonium odoratissimum)*

FORM: Capsules, teas, and tablets

HERBAL PROPHYLAXIS AND TREATMENT:

Prevention: Insure that a strict and sanitary hygiene is maintained. Use **antimicrobial herbs**: Take one capsule three times a day, three times a week (every other day) or one cup of tea made from any three-herb mixture, three times a week (every other day) for one to two weeks prior to traveling in an endemic diphtheria area or during an outbreak.

Treatment: Drink copious amounts of various fluids daily for their rehydration effect throughout the course of the illness and convalescence. Take **antitoxin herbs (goldenseal, gentian, bayberry, and lemongrass)** and **antimicrobial herbs:** Take two to three capsules three times a day or one cup of tea made from any three-herb mixture three times a day for one week, then rotate combination of herbs each week until symptoms are gone. Follow additional treatment instruction found in this section.

- With diphtheria the throat area should be cleared of the phlegm and false mucous membrane using a **bayberry** and **raspberry** combination and **garlic.**
- A mouthwash solution of **goldenseal** and **myrrh,** with a small amount of **ginger,** may be used as a gargle every half hour to clear the mucus and germ out of the throat.
- Continue taking antimicrobial herbs throughout the course of this disease.
- Antispasmodic herbal agents such as **lobelia, skullcap, black cohosh, anise seed, peppermint, fennel, cramp bark, licorice,** and **chamomile** provide relief while warding off the dangers of paralysis.
- A purified type of **turpentine** (found in most pharmacies) used as a fomentation to the throat and a **cayenne** fomentation on the chest and the lung area can be beneficial.
- One should always give an emetic (to stimulate vomiting) before allowing the patient to go to sleep, and the bowels should be cleansed of poisons with high enemas accompanied with stimulant herbs. Any of the following herbs may be used for enemas: **bayberry bark, raspberry leaves, catnip, chickweed, white oak bark, shepherd's purse, wild alum root, echinacea, strawberry leaves.**
- The patient should be encouraged to drink plenty of water to flush the kidneys of toxic products.
- A hot steam bath and a hot foot bath of **mustard** (given alternately) are beneficial. Also, a fomentation of **mullein** and **ragwort** may be applied to the throat for their soothing properties.
- Hydrotherapy (wet sheet pack) can be used for fever symptoms, especially during the night. See Appendix for instructions.
- Other hot and cold fomentations can be given over the liver, stomach, kidneys, and spine to keep the circulation normal. This stimulates the lymphatic system, helps clean out toxins, and provides a precaution against paralysis.
- If the heart rate is rapid, apply an ice bag over the heart.
- In case of headache, place cold compresses or ice bags to the head and neck.
- **Bayberry bark** or **lemon juice** will relieve the soreness in the throat.
- Heavy food intact should be avoided during the course of the illness. Have patient drink ample fresh **pineapple juice, carrot juice, citrus**

juice, and other fresh juices and broths until a nutritious plant-based diet can be tolerated.

• Where one suspects a light attack, a gargle of **white oak bark** with a little **ginger** will arrest further development.

• Apply tincture of **cayenne** around the neck, then cover with flannel material for a fomentation.

• Infuse **sumac berries** for one-half hour in water, strain and sweeten to taste with a small amount of honey, then mix with fresh **pineapple juice**; use this as a gargle.

• One or two enemas should be given daily to keep the bowels clear.

• If properly cared for, the disease will end within 7 to 10 days.

• Each day, clean all clothing and bed linen by boiling or disinfecting.

CONTRAINDICATIONS: None

HEPATITIS

Infectious hepatitis is an acute inflammation of the liver. It may be caused by a virus, bacterium, or toxic substance. There are six viral types of hepatitis (A, B, C, D, E, G). Our discussion is limited to two strains caused by viruses hepatitis A and hepatitis B.

Hepatitis A is usually transmitted via food, milk, and water contaminated with infected fecal matter and is most common in areas where sanitation is poor. The incubation period is 15 to 45 days. Hepatitis A is nearly always a self-limiting disease with a complete recovery usual and a low mortality rate (less than 0.2 percent). The person with hepatitis is most infectious just before the onset of symptoms. Very occasionally the case is fulminating, with delirium, high fever, and intense jaundice, and without correct treatment these cases may be fatal.

Hepatitis B is also known as serum hepatitis and is contracted via inadequately sterilized syringes and needles, poor surgical techniques, and sexual contact. The incubation period is three to six months. High-risk groups for contracting hepatitis B are intravenous drug users, the sexually promiscuous, and healthcare workers who handle bodily fluids.

Some countries have instated a routine hepatitis B vaccination schedule for all children, regardless of whether or not they are at a high risk of contracting the disease. Other countries have suspended hepatitis B vaccinations because of fears the vaccine could cause neurological disorders, particularly multiple sclerosis.

The symptoms of hepatitis develop over a few days, including fatigue, headache, irritability, joint stiffness, vomiting, nausea, stomach pain, diarrhea or constipation, muscle ache, fever, itching or skin rashes, and a loss of appetite. Nausea, especially at the sight of food and particularly fatty food, is a complaint. After a few days of these symptoms, the urine becomes dark and the feces pale. The conjunctiva of the eyes and the skin become yellow as jaundice develops.

Even those with only a mild case of hepatitis should rest in bed, as this lessens the damage to the liver and hastens recovery. The diet must be very light with no fats and no alcohol. Alcohol, drugs, and rich foods should be avoided for many months following hepatitis to allow the liver to recover. Professional treatment is advised, particularly in severe cases. Immunization is not advised for pregnant women.

HERBALS AND BOTANICALS: **Astragalus** *(Astragalus membranaceus)*, **Barberry** *(Berberis vulgaris)*, **Blessed Thistle** *(Cnicus benedictus)*, **Dandelion Root** *(Taraxacum officinale)*, **Fennel Seed** *(Foeniculum vulgare)*, **Goldenseal** *(Hydrastis Canadensis)*, **Grapefruit Seed Extract, Lemon Balm** *(Melissa officinalis)*, **Licorice** *(Glycyrrhiza glabra)*, **Milk Thistle** *(Silybum marianum)*, **Oregon Grape** *(Mahonia aquifolium)*, **Peppermint** *(Mentha x piperita)*, **Schisandra** *(Schisandra chinensis)*, **St. John's Wort** *(Hypericum perforatum)*, **Turmeric** *(Curcuma longa)*, **Skullcap** *(Scutellaria lateriflora)*, **Yarrow** *(Achillea millefolium)*

FORM: Capsules, teas, and tablets

HERBAL PROPHYLAXIS AND TREATMENT:
Prevention: Avoid contaminated water, milk, or food, and avoid toxic substances, poisonous chemicals, fumes, and drugs of all kind. Healthcare personnel should maintain caution when handling bodily fluids. Insure that a strict and sanitary hygiene is maintained. Use **liver detoxifiers/antiviral herbs (barberry, blessed thistle, dandelion root, goldenseal, grapefruit seed extract, lemon balm, licorice, milk thistle, Oregon grape, schisandra, St. John's wort)** and other **antimicrobial herbs:** Take one capsule three times a day, three times a week (every other day) or one cup of tea made from any three-herb mixture, three times a week (every other day) for one to two weeks prior to traveling in a high-risk hepatitis area or during an outbreak.

Treatment: Insure that a strict and sanitary hygiene is maintained. Drink copious amounts of various fluids daily to keep kidneys flushed throughout the course of the illness and convalescence. Take **antitoxin herbs (goldenseal, gentian, bayberry, lemongrass)** and the **antimicrobial herbs** until symptoms disappear. Take two to three capsules three times a day or one cup of tea made from any three-herb mixture three times a day for one week, then rotate combination of herbs each week until symptoms are gone. Follow the other herbal agent recommendations and instructions given in the treatment procedures.

- Most cases of hepatitis are self-limiting and will heal with rest and supportive care. Bed rest has been considered important in the treatment of hepatitis in the past. Specialists believe that the fatigue which accompanies the disease will limit the amount of exercise the patient feels up to participating in; they should be encouraged to exercise but avoid becoming overly tired.
- The patient often has a poor appetite, and sometimes even the smell of food cooking will cause nausea. Helping the patient receive adequate nourishment is often a challenge. Be sure the patient receives a nutritious breakfast, as hepatitis patients tend to lose their appetites as the day wears on. Avoid heavy, greasy foods and alcoholic beverages. An oil-free diet is recommended.
- Constipation should be guarded against, as accumulations of stool in the large bowel allow the bloodstream to absorb more waste products such as ammonia, increasing the workload of the inflamed liver.
- **Carrot juice** (6 to 8 ounces) twice a day is helpful in healing the liver.
- Alternating **castor oil** and **burdock leaf** packs applied over the liver can relieve discomfort and inflammation.
- The patient should be encouraged to drink plenty of water to flush the kidneys of toxic products.
- The patient should bathe frequently and be careful to wash the hands with soap and warm water after every bowel movement. It is best for the patient to have a separate toilet, but if this is not possible, wash the toilet seat after each use.
- The patient should not prepare food for others or be in the food preparation area and should use disposable eating utensils if possible; if not, utensils should be washed separately from those of the rest of the family. Disposable eating utensils should be placed in plastic bags for disposal.
- Linen and personal clothing should be laundered separately.
- The hepatitis patient should be protected from toxic fumes, such as cleaning liquids.
- Drugs for hepatitis should be kept to a minimum, as these substances are toxic to the liver. There are no antibiotics available to combat hepatitis. Birth control pills containing estrogens are known to raise the serum bilirubin levels and should not be taken. Corticosteroids given during the acute phase may lead to later relapse, and they provide no demonstrable benefit. Even aspirin is toxic to the liver.

- The following herbs help the liver regenerate: **barberry, blessed thistle, dandelion root, goldenseal, grapefruit seed extract, lemon balm, licorice, milk thistle, Oregon grape, schisandra, St. John's wort.**
- Use the antimicrobial herbs to treat or check possible secondary infection throughout the course of this disease.
- Hot fomentations over the liver area for 15 to 20 minutes, followed by a cold sponging, repeating the alternating hot and cold four times, may be done on a daily basis. Finish the treatment with a shower or sponge bath.
- A charcoal and flaxseed poultice over the liver may be used at night to detoxify and heal the liver.
- A hot bath may be given to raise the body temperature and assist the body in fighting the virus. The patient sits in a tub of water as hot as can be tolerated until the body temperature reaches 102 to 104° F. The water temperature may then be cooled to maintain this body temperature for approximately 20 minutes. Apply washcloths wrung from ice water to the face and head to keep the head cool. Give the patient plenty of water to drink, as he will lose fluids through perspiration. After 20 minutes give a cool shower, dress the patient warmly, and have him rest in bed until the sweating stops. The treatment may be given for 10 to 15 days, but some patients may not be able to tolerate the physical taxation of daily treatments.
- Adequate bed rest lessens damage to liver, and fever therapy hastens recovery.

CONTRAINDICATIONS: None

INFLUENZA (FLU)

Influenza is a viral infection of the intestinal or respiratory tract, which is often accompanied by symptoms of aching and feverishness. Different strains of influenza will cause different symptoms, including sore throats, coughs, and gastric disorders. This epidemic affliction is characterized by catarrhal inflammation of the mucous membranes of the throat and bronchi, accompanied by mucopurulent discharge, fever, vascular prostration, and severe neuralgia pains. Complications of pleurisy and neuritis may appear. Symptoms come on about 48 hours after exposure.

Influenza virus is basically airborne and most commonly spread by droplets containing the virus. The infected droplets are spread by coughing, sneezing, kissing, and the use of drinking glasses, towels, or other contaminated articles.

Influenza normally lasts from two to five days, but more serious complications can develop, particularly in the elderly. There seems to be an increasing tendency for influenza symptoms to linger, leaving the person feeling debilitated and depressed afterwards.

Immunization is carried out, particularly on the elderly, at the beginning of the winter. Because there are so many different strains of influenza, the effectiveness is very limited. Flu vaccines can also act as a trigger for asthma[74] and visual disorders.[75]

HERBALS AND BOTANICALS: Astragalus *(Astragalus membranaceus)*, **Bugleweed** *(Lycopus virginicus)*, **Cat's Claw** *(Uncaria tomentosa)*, **Celery Seed** *(Apium graveolens)*, **Cinchona Bark** *(Cinchona spp.)*, **Echinacea** *(Echinacea purpurea)*, **Elderberry** *(Sambucus nigra.)*, **Eucalyptus** *(Eucalyptus globulus)*, **Garlic** *(Allium sativum)*, **Ginger** *(Zingiber offinicinale)*, **Goldenrod** *(Solidago virgaurea)*, **Goldenseal** *(Hydrastis canadensis)*, **Lemongrass** *(cymbopogon citratus)*, **Licorice Root** *(Glycyrrhiza glabra)*, **Lobelia** *(Lobelia inflata)*, **Marshmallow Root** *(Althaea officinalis)*, **Pau d'Arco** *(Tabebuia avellanedae)*, **Pennyroyal** *(Mentha pulegium)*, **Peppermint** *(Mentha x piperita)*, **Plantain** *(Plantago major)*, **Sage** *(Salvio officinalis)*, **Siberian Ginseng** *(Eleutherococcus senticosus/Acanthopanax senticosus)*, **Slippery Elm** *(Ulmus rubra)*, **Black Walnut** *(Juglans nigra)*, **White Willow Bark** *(Salix alba)*, **Wormwood** *(Artemisia absinthium)*, **Yarrow** *(Achillea millefolium)*

FORM: Capsules, teas, and tablets

HERBAL PROPHYLAXIS AND TREATMENT:

Prevention: Be careful to prevent influenza. It can become serious very rapidly. Insure that a strict and sanitary hygiene is maintained. Use **antimicrobial herbs:** Take one capsule three times a day, three times a week (every other day) or one cup of tea made from any three-herb mixture, three times a week (every other day) for one to two weeks prior to traveling in an endemic influenza area or during an outbreak.

Treatment: Treat influenza aggressively. It is becoming serious when the voice becomes hoarse, pain develops in the chest, and when yellow or green phlegm is brought up. Use **antimicrobial herbs:** Take two to three capsules three times a day or one cup of tea made from any three-herb mixture three times a day for one week, then rotate combination of herbs each week until symptoms are gone. Follow the other herbal agent recommendations and instructions given in the treatment procedures below. Drink copious amounts of various fluids daily to reduce the amount of mucus throughout the course of the illness and convalescence. Get adequate rest.

- Antibiotics do not have any significant beneficial effect on the influenza virus and should not be used.
- The antimicrobial herbs may be used throughout the course of this disease.
- Increase fluid intake. Drink at least 10 glasses of water a day to help keep secretions in the lungs thin.
- For sore throat that sometimes accompanies flu, gargle (see Notes on Hydrotherapy in the Appendix) for 10 minutes every two to four hours using hot salty water: one teaspoon salt in one pint of warm water.
- A humidifier or steam inhalations may be helpful if there is chest congestion or nasal stuffiness. A regular lamp with a 60-watt bulb held one to two inches from the nose for periods of five minutes is a great help for nasal stuffiness.
- **Eucalyptus** as a vapor works well to relieve congestion.
- Herbal teas of **peppermint, elderberry or flower, pennyroyal, fresh ginger,** and **fresh garlic** may also be used to relieve congestion. During the convalescent period, **cat's claw, celery, goldenrod, lobelia, plantain, sage, slippery elm,** and **white willow bark** may be useful for their diuretic, anti-inflammatory, antispasmodic, and immune-enhancing effect.
- Irrigating the nasal cavities and gargling with warm salt water may minimize or prevent influenza virus from causing illness. Some researchers believe irrigation diminishes the likelihood of the influenza virus lodging in the nose.
- Use warm, close-fitting bed clothes, laundered daily during the acute phase. It is important to dress properly to avoid the slightest chilling, while avoiding overdressing, which might induce sweating. Viruses grow well in a warm environment.
- Hot fomentations to the chest may aid congestion.
- Hot foot baths may assist in relieving headaches and nasal congestion.
- A contrast shower can be used to enhance the function of the immune system.
- Back rubs may be given as a comfort measure and to activate the immune and lymphatic systems.
- The room should have a good supply of fresh air at all times, but no draft on the patient should be permitted. A draft is identified when

the patient's skin becomes cooler than the forehead or when the patient experiences discomfort. Actually compare the forehead temperature with that of the backs of the arms, the earlobes, ankles, and so on.

- Take an enema at the first symptoms. The bowels should be kept clear with **senna tea**, as respiratory viruses are shed partially through the gastrointestinal tract.
- Do not smoke. Influenza occurs 21 percent more frequently in smokers than in non-smokers.
- Use a sugar-free, low-fat diet to prevent weakening of the immune system.
- A deep breathing exercise may be done every two hours or any time the patient thinks of it. Take a deep breath, hold for a slow count of 20, exhale through the nose, and hold breath out for a count of 10. Repeat 30 to 50 times. This procedure refreshes blood flow to the tissue of the upper respiratory passages, carries away wastes, and encourages healing.
- **Lemongrass:** Citral is the principle constituent of lemongrass oil. This substance kills even the most acute influenza viruses and is effective for all fever-induced diseases.

CONTRAINDICATIONS: None

MALARIA

Four species of the malarial parasite infect man, and they are all carried by mosquitoes of the genus *Anopheles*, which flourish in tropical and subtropical countries.

The risk of contracting malaria varies according to the season and locality. The most effective way to avoid malaria is to prevent being bitten by mosquitoes. Wear protective clothing, use insect repellents, and sleep under a mosquito net.

The main symptoms of malaria are headaches, chills, and fevers (shivering fit). Jaundice and general malaise may develop. A blood test should be taken to confirm diagnosis. Most common is "benign" malaria which is characterized by intermittent fevers that may recur from time to time for several years. The mortality rate of benign malaria in previously healthy people is low. "Malignant" malaria, which is more common in West Africa, although it is also found elsewhere, is characterized by profound jaundice and profound anemia, and urgent professional treatment must be sought, as the mortality rate of this type of malaria is high.

Orally administered drugs are the orthodox technique for attempting to avoid malaria. The malarial parasites are increasingly resistant to these drugs, and they should not be taken during pregnancy. Antimalarial drugs can also cause a number of well-reported side effects, including drowsiness, headaches, visual disturbances, and tinnitus. For more information, the World Health Organization produces a useful fact sheet.

HERBALS AND BOTANICALS: Boneset (*Eupatorium perfoliatum*), **Quinine** (*Cinchona officinalis*), **Echinacea** (*Echinacea augustifolia, E. pallida, E. purpura*), **Elderberry and Flowers** (*Sambucus nigra*), **Garlic** (*Allium sativum*), **Gentian Root** (*Gentiana lutea*), **Goldenseal** (*Hydrastis Canadensis*), **Lemongrass** (*Cymbopogon citratus*), **Meadowsweet** (*Filipendula ulmaria*), **Neem** (*Azadirachta indica*), **Pau d'Arco** (*Tabebuia avellanedae*), **Peppermint** (*Mentha x piperita*), **Quassia Bark** (*Picrasma excelsa*), **Schisandra** (*Schisandra chinensis*), **Senna** (*Senna alexandrina*), **Sweet Annie** (*Artemisia annua*), **White Willow Bark** (*Salix alba, S. cinereas*), **Wormwood** (*Artemisia absinthium*)

FORM: Capsule, teas, and tablets

HERBAL PROPHYLAXIS AND TREATMENT:
   Prevention: Insure that strict measures are taken to prevent mosquito bites. Use **anti-malarial herbs (artemisia or Sweet Annie, astragalus, black adler bark, cinchona bark, gentian root, neem tree, quassia bark, white willow bark)** and **antimicrobial herbs:** Take one capsule three times a day, three times a week (every other day) or one cup of tea made from any three-herb mixture, three times a week (every other day) for one to two weeks prior to traveling in an endemic mosquito area. The best protection from malaria is to prevent mosquito bites and control mosquito breeding environment; use screens, netting with impregnated repellants, and insecticides over bed.

- Mosquito repellents: Aromatic herbs used inside the house, **African marigold or** *Tagetes erecta, Tageta minuta,* **lemongrass,** *Artemisia annua* are helpful.
- Eating one to two cloves of raw **garlic** a day acts as a skin repellant for mosquitoes.
- Eight to 10 drops of **Grapefruit Seed Extract (GSE)** three times a day or tablets equal to 10 to 15 drops of GSE may be used for prevention.

Treatment: Drink (especially during fever) copious amounts of various fluids daily for their rehydration effect throughout the course of the illness and convalescence. **Take antitoxin herbs (goldenseal, gentian, bayberry, lemongrass) and antimalarial herbs (artemisia or Sweet Annie, astragalus, black adler bark, cinchona bark, gentian root, neem tree, quassia bark, white willow bark).** Other **antimicrobial herbs** may be used for secondary infections: Take two to three capsules three times a day or one cup of tea made from any three-herb mixture three times a day for one week, then rotate combination of herbs each week until symptoms are gone.

- A vegetarian diet is important; it should be rich in vegetables and fresh fruits, especially those high in vitamin C, such as **lemons, bitter oranges, kiwis, pineapples, mangoes,** and **papayas.**
- Drink plenty of fluids, water, natural juices, potassium-rich broths, and vegetable broth. These should be cool, not cold.
- **Charcoal** poultices may be helpful for painful joints, as well as the enlarged liver and spleen.
- **Gentian root** destroys the protozoa that cause malaria; **cinchona bark** is antimalarial and decreases fever.
- A well-timed hydrotherapy treatment can benefit all malaria patients. The treatment should be timed to the cycles of fever, since the temperature will usually go up at the same time each day and in the same cycle (such as every four hours). General revulsive fomentation over the liver and spleen with two minutes of cold mitten friction should be used. A hot and cold contrast shower at the beginning of symptoms may reduce symptoms. The shower should be three minutes of hot followed by 30 seconds of cold for four changes. Have the patient rest for at least 30 minutes following treatment. Note: If daily chills begin, note the time of day and take a hot and cold shower or steam treatment 30 minutes before onset on subsequent days.
- For high fevers (above 104° F.) mild hydrotherapy may reduce the temperature. A wet sheet pack with a cool cloth to the head may alleviate chills; apply for 20 minutes. A cool water enema may also bring the temperature down. Be sure to keep patient well hydrated. Oral rehydration treatments will afford some hydration.
- The antimicrobial herbal agents may be used throughout the course of this disease.
- **Artemisia or Sweet Annie, black adler bark, catnip, meadowsweet,** and **quassia bark** may be used to decrease fever.
- **Elderberry** may be used for feverish chills.

CONTRAINDICATIONS: None

MEASLES (RUBEOLA)

Measles is a highly contagious classic childhood illness. The early symptoms are sore throat, cold symptoms, inflamed eyes, cough, nasal drainage, itching, and feverishness. On about the fourth day a rash appears on the child's neck and behind the ears, which gradually moves downward to cover the body. Most children recover fully without treatment after about 10 days. The incubation period is 10 to 12 days, and the most infectious period is just before the rash appears. The virus is spread by droplet spray from the mouth, throat, and nose.

In the vast majority of children who catch measles, the disease disappears and the only aftereffect is lifelong immunity to another attack. Very occasionally complications develop, usually caused by dehydration from a high fever or by difficulty breathing due to a secondary chest infection. Contrary to the popular myth, there is no danger of permanent eye damage except in malnourished children when vitamin A is deficient. Extremely rarely, a more serious complication involving inflammation of the brain tissues (encephalitis) may develop. Seek urgent medical treatment if there are any signs of unusual drowsiness, a severe headache, or marked irritability. Encephalitis is most likely to result from "atypical" measles, which is more common in children immunized against measles. Other complications can usually be handled by very vigorous application of simple remedies and are nearly always prevented by the treatment methods described below.

In 1994 a study showed a possible connection between the measles inoculation and the sharp rise in Crohn's disease and colitis in children.[76] The measles vaccine has also been known to cause deaths from infection, thrombocytopenia, and fatal shock, and in a Danish study the vaccine was linked to arthritis and dermatitis.

Studies as far back as 1991 show that some children vaccinated for measles develop allergic hypersensitivity reactions.[77]

HERBALS AND BOTANICALS: Amur Corktree (*Phellodendron amurense*), **Calendula flower** (*Calendula officinalis*), **Catnip** (*Nepeta cataria*), **Chamomile** (*Matricaria recututa*), **Chickweed** (*Stellaria media*), **Cleavers** (*Galium aparine*), **Coltsfoot** (*Tussilago farfara*), **Echinacea** (*Echinacea purpurea*), **Eucalyptus** (*Eucalyptus spp.*), **Forsythia** (*Forsythia suspense*), **Fireflame Bush** (*Woodfordia floribunda*), **Gentian** (*gentiana lutea*), **Goldthread** (*Coptis chinensis*), **Horehound** (*Marrubium vulgare L.*), **Kosam Seed** (*Brucea javanica*), **Licorice** (*Glycyrrhiza glabra*), **Mugwort** (*Artemisia princes*), **Mullein** (*Verbascum thapsus*), **Saffron** (*Caesalpinia sappan*), **Pleurisy Root** (*Asclepias tuberosa*), **Pomegranate** (*Punica granatum*), **Raspberry Leaves** (*Rubus idaeus*), **Red Sage** (*Salvia officinalis* var. *rubia*), **Spicebush**

(*Lindera benzoin*), **Thyme** *(Thymus vulgaris),* **Japanese Sumac** *(Rhus javanica),* **Chinese Skullcap** *(Scutellaria-baicalensis),* **Valarian** *(Valerian officinalis),* **Wax Tree** *(Rhus succedanea* L.*)*, **Witch Hazel** *(Hamamelis virginiana),* **Yarrow** *(Achillea millefolium)*

FORM: Capsules, teas, and tablets

HERBAL PROPHYLAXIS AND TREATMENT:
    Prevention: Avoid outbreak area unless you want to be exposed to acquire lifelong immunity (it is very contagious). Insure that a strict and sanitary hygiene is maintained. Use **antimicrobial herbs:** Take one capsule three times a day, three times a week (every other day) or one cup of tea made from any three-herb mixture, three times a week (every other day) for one to two weeks prior to traveling in an endemic measles area or during an outbreak.
    Treatment: Use **antiviral/antimicrobial herbs:** Take two to three capsules three times a day or one cup of tea made from any three-herb mixture three times a day for one week, then rotate combination of herbs each week until symptoms are gone.

- Antibiotics should be strictly avoided, as they do not influence the course of the measles or decrease the rate of complications from measles but do add another injurious agent for the body to fight.
- The antimicrobial herbs may be used throughout the course of this disease.
- Fluids should be encouraged, particularly during fever. The mouth may be rather sore, therefore bland drinks and food may be soothing.
- There is no proof that light is injurious to vision, but the patient may be sensitive to light and more comfortable in darkened room. An eye wash made of **eyebright** or a compress of **chamomile** will ease the discomfort of photosensitivity.
- Saline compresses applied to the eyes may be soothing. Use one teaspoon of salt to one pint of water to make a normal saline solution.
- Cool moisture from a vaporizer may greatly reduce any cough.
- Itching may be treated with **olive oil** or **aloe gel** rubbed into the skin. Also, corn starch or oatmeal baths may be soothing. **Chickweed** has been used for its anti-itching effect. **Witch hazel** applied to the skin will usually provide immediate but temporary relief.
- Water given copiously is the best cough medicine. Yet **horehound, licorice, coltsfoot,** and **mullein** will help both the cough and sooth the sore throat.

- A hot bath treatment may help relieve the fever. Place the child in a tub of hot water (104 to 108° F.) about one minute for each year of his age. Be careful to keep the head cool. The treatment may be repeated every two hours. After treatment, dress the patient warmly to prevent chilling.
- **Garlic** and **catnip** enemas are helpful in decreasing fever; tea made from **catnip, linden,** and **yarrow** is especially appropriate for reducing fever.
- The other herbs mentioned at the beginning of this section are helpful for the various symptoms of measles.
- Hot fomentations to the chest may be helpful for the bronchioles. Fomentations may also be used twice a day, accompanied by a hot foot bath. A heating compress can be applied overnight.
- Hot foot baths may also be used for headache.
- A plant-based diet is best, while avoiding processed foods.

CONTRAINDICATIONS: None

MENINGITIS

Meningitis is an inflammation of the membranes (*meninges*) that surround the brain and the spinal cord. There are two types of meningitis, viral and bacterial. Viral meningitis is normally much milder than bacterial meningitis and can often be mistaken for a bad case of flu. It usually clears up on its own within a week or two. But the bacterial type requires prompt, aggressive treatment or brain damage or death can result. (Any time a bacterial infection in the head or throat occurs [such as strep throat or an ear infection] eliminate it; do not ignore the problem.)

Symptoms of meningitis, which may appear suddenly, often include high fever, severe and persistent headache, stiff neck, nausea, general malaise, shivering, intolerance of light, drowsiness, irritability, and vomiting. They may be associated with a throat or ear infection or with cold symptoms that then rapidly deteriorate. Changes in behavior such as confusion, sleepiness, and difficulty waking up are extremely important symptoms and may require emergency treatment. In infants, symptoms of meningitis may include irritability or tiredness, poor feeding, and fever. There are currently two different vaccinations offered routinely for two different strains of bacterial meningitis: haemophilus influenzae type B (Hib) and meningitis C.

The Hib bacterium is present in the nasal mucus of most people and doesn't cause any problems in a healthy person. Once Hib disease is activated it can cause symptoms of meningitis and septicemia.

Hib disease is most common in preschool children, with the highest incidence in infants between six and 11 months of age. It has been observed that the incidence is far higher among children in daycare centers and primary schools, particularly among non-toilet trained children in daycare.

HERBALS AND BOTANICALS: **Catnip** *(Nepeta cataria)*, **Echinacea** *(Echinacea purpurea)*, **Garlic** *(Allium sativum)*, **Goldenseal** *(Hydrastis canadensis)*, **Grapefruit Seed Extract**, **St. Johns Wort** *(Hypericum perforattum)*, **Lobelia** *(Lobelia inflata)*, **Olive Leaf Extract** *(Olea europaea)*

FORM: Capsules, teas, and tablets

HERBAL PROPHYLAXIS AND TREATMENT:
Prevention: Keep the immune system working optimally and avoid immune-suppressing lifestyle practices and drugs. Insure that a strict and sanitary hygiene is maintained. Use **antimicrobial herbs:** Take one capsule three times a day, three times a week (every other day) or one cup of tea made from any three-herb mixture, three times a week (every other day) for one to two weeks prior to traveling in an endemic meningitis area or during an outbreak.
Treatment: Meningitis requires rapid diagnosis and initiation of treatment. Treat head/face and upper respiratory infection promptly and aggressively. Drink copious amounts of various fluids daily for their rehydration effect throughout the course of the illness and convalescence. Use **antimicrobial herbs:** Take two to three capsules three times a day or one cup of tea made from any three-herb mixture three times a day for one week, then rotate combination of herbs each week until symptoms are gone.

- It is wise to seek prompt diagnosis and treatment for a bacterial or viral infection.
- If cerebral meningitis: Immerse back of head in warm Epsom salt solution several times daily to draw out inflammation. Alternate hot and cold packs on the neck and back of head to stimulate circulation to the area, plus fomentations to the liver and abdomen.
- If spinal meningitis: Give fomentation to the spine, liver, and abdomen.
- The bowels must move two to three times a day. Use herbal laxatives if necessary.
- If there is fever, take sponge baths. Use **lobelia** and **catnip** to reduce fever. **Catnip** may be used for an anal enema to reduce fever.

- **Lobelia** is very helpful in meningitis. Use in very small doses. When frequently given it will raise a vigorous perspiration, after which a long sleep of 10 to 12 hours may follow.
- **Echinacea, astragalus,** and **garlic** may be used for their immune-boosting properties.
- **Echinacea** and **goldenseal** are both good antibiotics. But do not take either one for more than a week; you can shift from one to the other. Take 6 to 8 **garlic** tablets or capsules daily.
- To strength nerves, take **skullcap** tea and **gota kola.**
- Avoid aspirin, which increases bleeding tendencies.
- Once the acute phase of the illness has passed and recovery has begun, eat a well-balanced vegetarian diet including fresh fruits and vegetables (at least 50 percent raw), grains, nuts, and seeds.
- Consume fresh **pineapple** and **papaya** frequently. Pineapples reduce inflammation; fresh papaya is good for digestion. Fresh fruits are the most effective.
- Other anti-inflammatory agents, such as **turmeric, rosemary,** and **ginger** may be used with good effect.
- Avoid all animal and dairy products, which encourage the formation of mucus. Avoid caffeine and processed foods, salt, sugar, and white flour products. A complete plant-based diet is recommended.
- Consider supplements: **Niacinamide** (100 to 500 mg daily), vitamin A (400 IU for children; 5,000 IU for adults), B complex, vitamin B6 (100 mg), vitamin B12 (2,000 mcg), **choline** (500 mg). Vitamin C (one-half teaspoon every hour during acute phase; reduce by half for maintenance until remission).
- Rest in bed in a dimly lit and well-ventilated room and drink plenty of water and high-nutrient liquids.
- The antimicrobial herbal agents may be used throughout the course of this disease.

CONTRAINDICATIONS: Do not take **goldenseal** internally on a daily basis for more than seven days, as it may disturb the normal intestinal flora. Do not use in large quantities during pregnancy, and use it with caution if allergic to ragweed.

MUMPS

Mumps is caused by a viral infection of the salivary glands (parotids) found in front of and below each ear. It is one of the common childhood diseases, characterized by swelling in one or both of the salivary glands. Other symptoms include feverishness and sore throat. No particular treatment is necessary, as mumps in children is not a serious illness. The swelling usually begins to go down after two or three days.

Currently the immunization against mumps is performed on infants as part of the MMR vaccine. This is promoted on the basis that although mumps is not a serious illness for children, it may cause orchitis, a swelling of the testicles, in adult men. There is a commonly held belief that mumps contracted by an adult male will result in sterility; this is actually extremely rare, as nearly all cases clear up totally, and usually only one testicle is affected.

It makes far more sense for boys to get mumps before they become adults, then sterility cannot occur. In fact, it is not known whether or not protection from the mumps vaccine lasts into adulthood, whereas having mumps as a child nearly always provides protection as an adult. According to the National Foundation for Infectious Diseases, 20 percent of the adults who get mumps are asymptomatic and nearly 50 percent have non-specific or primarily respiratory symptoms, with or without parotiditis. Adult management focuses on treatment of symptoms: low grade fever, chills, swelling, and tenderness in glands. The treatment procedure for adult onset mumps is effective.

The reported side effects of the MMR vaccine include allergic reactions, febrile seizures, nerve deafness, and more rarely, encephalitis.

HERBALS AND BOTANICALS: Calendula (*Calendula officinalis*), **Chamomile** (*Matricaria recutita*), **Comfrey** (*Symphytum officinale*), **Echinacea** (*Echinacea* spp.), **Elderberry** (*Sambucus nigra*), **Garlic** (*Allium sativum*), **Gentian** (*Gentiana lutea*), **Goldenseal** (*Hydrastis canadensis*), **Licorice** (*Glycyrrhiza Glabra*), **Marshmallow** (*Althaea officinalis*), **Mullein** (*Verbascum thapsus*), **Onion** (*Allium cepa*), **Peppermint** (*Mentha piperita*), **Pokeweed Root** (*Phytolacca americana*), **Sage** (*Salvia officinalis*), **Slippery Elm** (*Ulmus rubra*), **Wormwood** (*Artemisia absinthoum*), **Yarrow** (*Achillea millefolium*)

FORM: Capsules, teas, and tablets

HERBAL PROPHYLAXIS AND TREATMENT:
Prevention: Insure that a strict and sanitary hygiene is maintained. Adults should avoid outbreak area, especially if they have not contracted

the disease before age 40. It may affect the ovaries and testes, causing sterility. Use **antitoxin** and **antimicrobial herbs:** Take one capsule three times a day, three times a week (every other day) or one cup of tea made from any three-herb mixture, three times a week (every other day) for one to two weeks prior to traveling in an area of outbreak.

Treatment: Drink adequate amounts of liquids throughout the course of the illness and convalescence. Use **antitoxin** and **antimicrobial herbs**: Take two to three capsules three times a day or one cup of tea made from any three-herb mixture three times a day for one week, then rotate combination of herbs each week until symptoms are gone. Strictly follow all other treatment instructions.

- Fluid intake must be adequate to replace fluids lost due to fever and loss of appetite.
- Cold or warm compresses may be applied to the neck for pain relief.
- The diet should be simple, sugar-free, and fat-free. Spicy, irritating foods and those requiring a lot of chewing should be avoided.
- A tepid bath or a hot half bath may be given for fever.
- For orchitis, an ice bag or cold compress to the scrotum is helpful. A charcoal compress at night may be helpful in controlling inflammation. Some have found considerable relief in the use of alternating hot and cold sitz baths. The worst is usually over in two to four days, with subsidence of symptoms in a week or more. A physician can do little except prescribe painkillers, which may make one sicker.
- As long as glands are swollen, eat mostly fruits and vegetables that are juiced or softened. A vegetarian diet is superior and will be helpful in minimizing the pain of chewing. **Pokeweed root** can be given for discomfort of swollen neck glands.
- Anti-inflammatory and demulcent herbs may be helpful in alleviating pain and discomfort in the throat: **chamomile, yarrow, calendula, peppermint, marshmallow, licorice, slippery elm, comfrey.**
- Keep patient warm and dry; get plenty of rest.
- The following antimicrobials may be used throughout the course of this disease: **aloe, buchu, calendula, Chinese skullcap, cloves, echinacea, elderberry, eucalyptus, garlic, ginseng, goldenseal, grapefruit seed extract, Japanese honeysuckle, lemon balm, lemon juice, licorice, lomatium root, myrrh, olive leaf, osha root, peppermint, rosemary, sage, tea tree, thyme, mint family of herbs.**

CONTRAINDICATIONS: None

POLIO

Poliomyelitis is caused by a viral infection which specifically attacks nerve cells in the spinal cord. The virus grows in the intestinal tract and is excreted in the feces; the incubation period is seven to 14 days. Whereas polio is still a significant disease in areas where sanitation is neglected and hygiene is poor, in Western countries polio is now an extremely rare disease.

The early symptoms of poliomyelitis include a headache, sore throat, and stiffness of the neck and back. In most cases the disease progresses no further, and unless there is a polio epidemic it is often mistaken for flu. If the full-blown disease sets in on the fourth or fifth day, paralysis develops and proceeds to its full extent in about 36 hours. The paralysis usually affects the limbs, and the muscles become painful and tender, beginning to waste about three weeks after the onset of paralysis. If the muscles of respiration are affected, breathing may become hampered. Rarely polio may also affect the brain, causing encephalitis.

It is important that anyone suspected of having polio rests in bed, as paralysis is more likely to occur in muscles which are kept active. After about three weeks the muscles may be gradually moved, and most will begin to recover at this time. Most people make a full recovery from polio, although rare fatalities do occur due to pneumonia or circulatory collapse. Physiotherapy should be continued for up to six months, as muscle recovery can continue through this period.

The effectiveness of the polio immunization in reducing the incidence of polio is controversial. There were three polio epidemics in the U.S. in the 20th century; the first two declined when there was no treatment offered. In the late 1940s, the decline of the third epidemic was credited to the polio vaccine, although this has since been disputed.

In recent years the inoculation against polio is the most common cause of polio in the developed world. Also, polio is excreted in the stools of those just vaccinated for approximately six weeks afterward, and there have been a small number of cases of parents contracting polio after changing the diapers of recently immunized infants. There is no evidence that public swimming pools spread polio in this way, most likely because the chlorine or other disinfectants in the water kill the virus.

As the vaccine is cultured in monkey kidney tissue, one of the unforeseen side effects has been transmission of the tumor-causing SV40 monkey virus. During the 1950s and 60s, tissue from SV40-infected monkeys was used in the vaccines. Millions of people have been inoculated with the polio vaccine contaminated with the tumoral virus SV40, and molecular genetic studies show that the virus was originally present in monkeys. It is possible that it will take 20 years or more before the eventual harmful effects of this virus will manifest. The polio vaccine has been held responsible for cases of encephalitis and Guillain-Barre Syndrome, which causes paralysis. Polio vaccines also contain small amounts of a number of antibiotics, and those with a hypersensitivity to antibiotics should avoid the vaccine. The vaccine should not be given during pregnancy.

HERBALS AND BOTANICALS: Black Cohosh *(Cimicifuga racemosa)*, **Calendula Flower** *(Calendula officinalis)*, **Catnip** *(Nepeta cataria)*, **Dandelion Root** *(Taraxacum officinale)*, **Goldenseal** *(Hydrastis canadensis)*, **Licorice** *(Glycyrrhiza glabra)*, **Milk Thistle** *(Silybum marianum)*, **Prickly Ash Berry** *(Zanthoxylum americanum)*, **Red Clover** *(Trifolium pretense)*, **Skullcap** *(Scutellaria lateriflora)*, **Valerian Root** *(Valeriana officinalis)*, **Wild Cherry Bark** *(Prunus serotina)*, **White Willow Bark** *(Salix alba, S. purpurea, S. fragilis)*, **Yellow Dock** *(Rumex crispus)*

FORM: Capsules, teas, and tablets

HERBAL PROPHYLAXIS AND TREATMENT:
Prevention: Insure that a strict and sanitary hygiene is maintained. Eliminate sugary foods, colas, and soft drinks from diet, as they predispose to polio by injuring or weakening nerves. Avoid cold temperatures, especially in the summer months, since cold intensifies the injury to nerve tissue. Use **antiviral/antimicrobial herbs:** Take one capsule three times a day, three times a week (every other day) or one cup of tea made from any three-herb mixture, three times a week (every other day) for one to two weeks during an outbreak.

Treatment: Drink plenty of non-sugary liquid and take warm tub baths throughout the course of the illness and convalescence. Use **antiviral/antimicrobial herbs**: Take two to three capsules three times a day or one cup of tea made from any three-herb mixture three times a day for one week, then rotate combination of herbs each week until symptoms are gone. Follow the other treatment instructions faithfully.

- Keep patient warm and dry. Get plenty of rest.
- As soon as a patient comes down with polio, the standard medical routine is to place him in bed and observe him to see if polio develops. But what should be done is to place him immediately in a warm, full bathtub or, even better, give hot pack to all parts of the body.

- During the infectious stage, keep the diet high in protein and potassium in order to replace that which is lost because of tissue destruction.
- Fluid, caloric, and sodium intake should be increased because of the fever. Additional B vitamins are needed, along with vitamin A (carrot juice and/or 5,000 IU vitamin A) and vitamin C (2,000-5,000 mg or more).
- Give antispasmodic tinctures and teas, such as **skullcap, lobelia, black cohosh, gum myrrh, skunk cabbage.**
- **Skullcap** and **valerian** soothe the nerves and prevent rupture of small blood vessels.
- Eat a complete plant-based diet with plenty of fruits and vegetables.
- Give hot and cold fomentations to the spine, stomach, and liver, and give massage to the entire body.
- Take plenty of exercise in open air with a sunbath daily.
- Cleanse the colon by giving an enema with **lobelia** and **catnip**.
- The following antimicrobials may be used throughout the course of this disease: **aloe, buchu, calendula, Chinese skullcap, cloves, echinacea, elderberry, eucalyptus, garlic, ginseng, goldenseal, grapefruit seed extract, Japanese honeysuckle, lemon balm, lemon juice, licorice, lomatium root, myrrh, olive leaf, osha root, peppermint, rosemary, sage, tea tree, thyme, mint family of herbs.**

CONTRAINDICATIONS: None

RUBELLA (GERMAN MEASLES)

Rubella, or German measles, is a harmless disease in children causing symptoms of slight feverishness, nasal discharge, and a rash of small, slightly raised spots that tend to move down the body. The duration is about three days or less. It is often called "three-day measles." Incubation period is from 14 to 21 days.

Rubella is less contagious than rubeola, and many children escape the disease, entering young adulthood without immunity, and females are thus able to contract the disease during pregnancy. Rubella is a potential threat to pregnant women, since those who contract it during the first three months of pregnancy are considered to have an approximately 10 percent risk of having a baby with birth defects, including blindness, deafness, a heart condition, cleft palate, or mental problems. It is for this reason that the inoculation is given to infants as part of the MMR injection. However, the immunity offered by inoculation does not last into adulthood, whereas contracting German measles as a child provides lifelong immunity. It would offer more protection to expose your daughter to German measles as a child.

Adults have relatively mild symptoms, including malaise, headache, joint stiffness, and lack of energy. Mild irritation of the nose and throat membranes may be present. Lymph node enlargement may occur. The rash, which begins on the face and neck and spreads to the trunk and extremities, may be the first indication of rubella. The rash lasts about three to four days and rarely itches.

For concerned women, a physician can order a blood test to check for natural immunity to rubella. Side effects to the MMR vaccine are well recorded, including convulsions, allergic reactions, and rarely, encephalitis.

HERBALS AND BOTANICALS: Boneset *(Eupatorium perfoliatum),* **Burdock Root** *(Arctium lappa),* **Calendula Flower** *(Calendula officinalis),* **Catnip** *(Nepeta cataria),* **Chamomile** *(Matricaria recutita),* **Elder Flower** *(Sambucus nigra),* **Garlic** *(Allium sativum),* **Goldenseal Root** *(Hydrastis canadensis),* **Hay Flower** *(Poa spp.),* **Licorice** *(Glycyrrhiza glabra),* **Peppermint** *(Mentha x piperita),* **Prickly Ash Berries** *(Zanthoxulum americanum),* **Red Clover** *(Trifolium pretense),* **White Willow Bark** *(Salix alba, Purpur, S. fragilis),* **Wild Cherry Bark** *(Salix alba, S. cinereas),* **Yellow Dock** *(Rumex crispus),* other herbs in **Mint** family may be used

FORM: Capsules, teas, and tablets

HERBAL PROPHYLAXIS AND TREATMENT:
Prevention: Avoid areas of outbreak. Expectant mothers must guard against exposure, as it is harmful to the fetus in the first trimester of pregnancy, possibly causing serious birth defects. Insure that a strict and sanitary hygiene is maintained. Use **antimicrobial herbs:** Take one capsule three times a day, three times a week (every other day) or one cup of tea made from any three-herb mixture, three times a week (every other day) for one to two weeks prior to traveling in an endemic area or during an outbreak.
Treatment: Drink copious amounts of various fluids daily for their rehydration effect throughout the course of the illness and convalescence. Avoid contact with others, especially children and adolescents. Take **antitoxin herbs (goldenseal, gentian, bayberry, lemongrass)** and **antimicrobial herbs**: Take two to three capsules three times a day or one cup of tea made from any three-herb mixture three times a day for one week, then rotate combination of herbs each week until symptoms and rash are gone.

- Use abundant fluids, water, fruit juices and vegetable broth, and a light diet free from added sugars and fats.
- A hot half bath may be used every two hours for fever or itching.
- If you need to lower the fever, **catnip** tea and **garlic** enemas will help. **Peppermint** tea is also good.
- A saline solution applied to the eyes is soothing, as is a darkened room.
- Salt water (or just plain hot water) gargles may be used for sore or irritated throat.
- Steam inhalations are useful if a cough is present.
- Isolate the patient to prevent further spread of the disease.
- If itching is present, a starch bath is often soothing. Add one cup of corn starch to about four inches of water in a bathtub. The patient may sit in the tub for 20 to 30 minutes and use a cup to dip the water onto the body parts not covered by the bath water. Pat dry to leave as much starch as possible on the skin.
- Ice bags may be applied to swollen neck glands for 5 to 15 minutes every hour if discomfort is severe.
- Herbal teas may be helpful: **catnip** tea for itching or irritability, **mint** tea for a stimulant if lethargic, and **red clover** tea as a general tonic.
- **Licorice** may be useful for the rubella virus. **Burdock, goldenseal,** and **yellow dock** will help to prevent secondary bacterial infections.
- **Boneset, chamomile, calendula,** and **white willow bark** will help with itching, irritability, and boosting the immune system.
- The following antimicrobials may be used throughout the course of this disease: **aloe, buchu, calendula, Chinese skullcap, cloves, echinacea, elderberry, eucalyptus, garlic, ginseng, goldenseal, grapefruit seed extract, Japanese honeysuckle, lemon balm, lemon juice, licorice, lomatium root, myrrh, olive leaf, osha root, peppermint, rosemary, sage, tea tree, thyme, mint family of herbs.**

CONTRAINDICATIONS: None

TETANUS

Tetanus (*Clostridium tetani*) is caused by bacteria which usually enter the body through wounds, especially deep penetrating wounds such as nail wounds. The bacillus is most commonly present in soil and especially in horse manure, so cleaning wounds thoroughly, particularly if infected with soil, is of the utmost importance in preventing the disease. Tetanus is extremely unlikely to develop from a wound that is washed thoroughly, kept clean, and exposed to air circulation.

The main symptoms of tetanus are severe muscular spasms that usually start in the jaw muscles, causing difficulty in opening the mouth (known as lockjaw). The spasms then spread to other muscles so that severe spasms become generalized. Orthodox treatment is to combine antibiotics, sedation, and curare with large doses of tetanus antitoxin. The mortality rate is about 10 percent.

Neither catching the disease nor the vaccination offer prolonged immunity. Thus, it would be more rational to vaccinate immediately following an incident with potential to cause tetanus, such as a deep wound or animal bite.

The tetanus immunization has caused death due to anaphylactic shock and also cases of Guillain-Barre Syndrome, which causes paralysis. It is given routinely to infants as part of the DTaP vaccine, and regular boosters are advised by the orthodox health system for adults.

HERBALS AND BOTANICALS: Black Cohosh (*Cimicifuga racemosa*), **Cramp Bark** (*Viburnum opulus*), **Lobelia** (*Lobelia inflata*), **Peach Leaf** (*Prunus persica*), **Senna** (*Senna Alexandrina*), **Skullcap** (*Scutellaria lateroflora*), **Skunk Cabbage** (*Symplocarpups foetidus*)

FORM: Capsules, teas, and tablets

HERBAL PROPHYLAXIS AND TREATMENT:
Prevention: Insure that a strict and sanitary hygiene is maintained. Take **antitoxin herbs (goldenseal, gentian, bayberry, lemongrass)** and **antimicrobial herbs**: Take one capsule three times a day, three times a week (every other day) or one cup of tea made from any three-herb mixture, three times a week (every other day) for one to two weeks prior to traveling.

Treatment: Drink copious amounts of various fluids daily for their rehydration effect throughout the course of the illness and convalescence. **Take antitoxin herbs (goldenseal, gentian, bayberry, lemongrass)** and **antimicrobial herbs:** Take two to three capsules three times a day or one cup of tea made from any three-herb mixture three times a day for one week, then rotate combination of herbs each week until symptoms are gone.

- Insure that any wound is thoroughly cleaned immediately after the incident. Hydrogen peroxide can be used. Deep penetrating wounds are of major concern.
- It is good practice to expose the wound to the direct rays of the sun several times a day.

- The following antimicrobials may be used throughout the course of this disease: **aloe, buchu, calendula, Chinese skullcap, cloves, echinacea, elderberry, eucalyptus, garlic, ginseng, goldenseal, grapefruit seed extract, Japanese honeysuckle, lemon balm, lemon juice, licorice, lomatium root, myrrh, olive leaf, osha root, peppermint, rosemary, sage, tea tree, thyme, mint family of herbs.**
- Mix two cups of **charcoal** or **wood ash** per gallon of water, then soak the limb or punctured part in it. If the wound is located where it cannot be soaked, apply the wood ash or charcoal solution in a fomentation. Do this for an hour and repeat if danger is suspected.
- A **peach leaf** poultice may be applied directly to the wound after washing. Change this raw poultice twice daily.
- A light plant-based diet should be given. Nourishing fresh fruit juices are especially helpful.
- Patient should be encouraged to drink freely of water (at least three quarts daily.)
- If patient is perspiring freely, a daily bath is indicated.
- A cathartic or laxative of **senna** should be given at the beginning of the sickness, and a daily laxative or cleansing enema may be indicated if bowel movements are not free.
- A general revulsive treatment to the abdomen should be repeated two or three times daily (see Notes on Hydrotherapy in the Appendix). Other hot and cold treatments can be used to combat infections located in the hands and limbs.
- Ice packs should be applied to the chest to protect the heart throughout illness.
- If a fever is present, use a tepid sponge bath with a cold compress to the head.
- Warm **purified turpentine** and apply to wound daily. Massage it over jaw, neck, and spine when symptoms of lockjaw are suspected.
- If lockjaw actually appears and the person shows stiffening, give antispasmodic tea (**black cohosh, cramp bark, lobelia, skullcap, skunk cabbage**) every 15 minutes until stiffening is gone.
- Keep patient warm and dry. Get plenty of rest.

CONTRAINDICATIONS: None

TUBERCULOSIS

Tuberculosis (TB) is caused by a highly contagious bacteria, *Mycobacterium tuberculosis*. There are two types that affect people: human and bovine types. The human type usually infects the lungs; the bovine type usually infects children and causes inflammation of the lymph glands and bones. The bovine type is spread by ingesting milk and has virtually disappeared due to improved public hygiene, the pasteurization of milk, and the prevention of tuberculosis in cattle.

The human type, also called pulmonary tuberculosis, is spread by infected sputum and by coughing. The most important single factor in the spread of pulmonary tuberculosis worldwide is overcrowded conditions; there is a direct correlation between an increase in the standard of living and a fall in the incidence of tuberculosis. Tuberculosis had virtually died out in the developed world; however, the past few years has seen a small increase in the number of cases, particularly in overcrowded neighborhoods of British inner cities.

Despite an active worldwide vaccination campaign, pulmonary tuberculosis is still prevalent in tropical countries, and the incidence is higher in recent immigrants from those parts of the world and in people who travel there. There also seems to be a link between TB and AIDS, as the groups with a high incidence of HIV and AIDS also have a high incidence of TB.

The effectiveness of the BCG vaccine varies greatly around the world, from zero to 80 percent. This variation is possibly due to strain variations, genetic or nutritional differences, and to environmental influences.[78] Side effects of the vaccine may include disseminated TB in immunosuppressed individuals, local ulceration, osteitis, lymphadenitis, and generalized lymphadenopathy.[79]

Symptoms of TB may be slow in developing and initially resemble those of influenza: general malaise, coughing, loss of appetite, night sweats, chest pain, and low grade fever. At first the cough may be nonproductive, but as the disease progresses, increasing amounts of sputum are produced. As the condition worsens, fevers, night sweats, chronic fatigue, weight loss, chest pain, and shortness of breath may occur, and the sputum may become bloody. In advanced cases, TB of the larynx can occur, making it impossible to speak above a whisper.

Orthodox treatment of TB is with a combination of antituberculous drugs. In the past few years, a number of TB strains have emerged that are resistant to antibiotics.

HERBALS AND BOTANICALS: Barberry *(Berberis vulgaris)*, **Butcher's Broom** *(Ruscus aculeatus)*, **Calendula** *(Calendula officinalis)*, **Cascara**

Segrada *(Rhamnus purshiana)*, **Cayenne** *(Capsicum annuum)*, **Chamomile** *(Matricaria recutita)*, **Comfrey** *(Symphytum officinale)*, **Echinacea** *(Echinacea* spp.*)*, **Eucalyptus** *(Eucalyptus globulus)*, **Elecampane** *(Inula helenium)*, **Forsythia** *(Forsythia suspensa)*, **Garlic** *(Allium sativum)*, **Goldenseal Root** *(Hydrastis canadensis)*, **Honeysuckle** *(Lonicera japonica)*, **Horehound** *(Marrubium vulgare)*, **Licorice** *(Glycyrrhiza glabra)*, **Lobelia** *(Lobelia inflata)*, **Marshmallow Root** *(Althaea officinalis)*, **Mullein** *(Verbascum thapsus)*, **Myrrh** *(Commiphora molmol)*, **Onion** *(Allium cepa)*, **Senna** *(Senna alexandrina)*, **Shepherd's Purse** *(Capsella bursa-pastoris)*, **Slippery Elm** *(Ulmus rubra)*, **Thyme** *(Thymus vulgaris)*, **Tamarisk** *(Tinospora cordifolia)*, **Yarrow** *(Achillea millefolium)*

FORM: Capsules, teas, and tablets

HERBAL PROPHYLAXIS AND TREATMENT:

Prevention: The basic formula for preventing TB is adequate rest, a good diet including calcium, and daily deep breathing outdoors. Use **antimicrobial herbs**: Take one capsule three times a day, three times a week (every other day) or one cup of tea made from any three-herb mixture, three times a week (every other day) for one to two weeks prior to traveling in an endemic tuberculosis area or during an epidemic.

Treatment: Drink copious amounts of various fluids daily for their rehydration effect throughout the course of the illness and convalescence. Take **antitoxin herbs (goldenseal, gentian, bayberry, lemongrass), antimicrobial herbs,** and other **herbs** recommended below in treatment instructions: Take two to three capsules three times a day or one cup of tea made from any three-herb mixture three times a day for one week, then rotate combination of herbs each week until symptoms are gone.

- Use abundant fluids and a light diet free from sugars and fats.
- To overcome the critical phase of this disease, fasting, rest, good food, and fresh air in the patient's room is very important.
- **Echinacea** is excellent for tuberculosis. Take two 450-mg capsules three times a day for a week; wait a week, then do it again. **Licorice** can be used during the alternate week. Another excellent remedy is **garlic**. Take one capsule three times a day or equivalent.
- Follow a plant-based diet with at least 50 percent raw fruits and vegetables. **Alfalfa sprouts, pomegranates, raw seeds** and **nuts, whole grains,** and **garlic** will promote healing.

- Drink fresh **pineapple, pomegranate, carrot** and **green** drinks. Also, **raw potato juice,** with compounds containing protease inhibitors, will aid recovery.
- Avoid stress. Rest, sunshine, and fresh air are most important for recovery.
- Individuals infected with TB should not use cortisone preparations. Cortisone suppresses immune function and makes the infection more difficult to treat and prevent.
- Vaccines and drugs cannot control TB if poor lifestyle practices are followed. Cleanliness and proper nutrition are vital in combating this disease.
- The following antimicrobials may be used throughout the course of this disease: **aloe, buchu, calendula, Chinese skullcap, cloves, echinacea, elderberry, eucalyptus, garlic, ginseng, goldenseal, grapefruit seed extract, Japanese honeysuckle, lemon balm, lemon juice, licorice, lomatium root, myrrh, olive leaf, osha root, peppermint, rosemary, sage, tea tree, thyme, mint family of herbs.**
- Maintain a moderate temperature and good ventilation in the sick room at all times. Prevent patient from becoming chilled.
- **Bayberry and shepherd's purse, bugleweed,** and **lobelia** will check hemorrhage of the lungs.
- Hot fomentations alternating with short cold applications should be applied to the front and back of chest. Also, give these along the full length of the spine and over the stomach, liver, and spleen. (See Notes on Hydrotherapy in the Appendix.)
- If a fever is present, a sponge bath with tepid water may be used. **Lemon juice** diluted in water will help break a fever. **Yarrow, red sage, catnip, peppermint, wild cherry bark, vervain, pleurisy root, nettle,** and **lobelia and red raspberry** tea are excellent for reduction of fever.
- It is helpful to keep bowels open with herbal laxatives such as **senna** or **cascara sagrada.**
- **Ginger, licorice, slippery elm, marshmallow,** and **mullein** can be used to sooth the throat and suppress coughing.
- To assist in cleansing pus and mucus accumulation, **comfrey, marshmallow, chickweed,** and **slippery elm** may be used every two hours. Remember, all sputum and discharges should be burned or buried.
- Get plenty of outdoor exercise and stay outdoors as much as possible.

CONTRAINDICATIONS: None

TYPHOID

Typhoid (enteric fever) is a disease of poor hygiene, being transmitted via the ingestion of contaminated food or water. It is most common in the tropics and subtropics. The disease organism affects the small intestine. While the symptoms are variable, they generally begin with a fever, and later severe diarrhea develops.

There are a number of possible complications of typhoid, including perforation of the intestine, pneumonia, meningitis, and inflammation of the gallbladder. Hospital treatment is advisable.

The efficacy of the immunization is not 100 percent, and immunity wears off after one to three years. Severe side effects to the inoculation are not uncommon, and it should not be performed on pregnant women, infants, or anyone suffering from an inflammatory illness, such as flu. Regular immunizations against typhoid can cause a hypersensitivity to the vaccine, and these people must also avoid further immunization.

HERBALS AND BOTANICALS: Blackberries *(Rubus villosus)*, **Black Cohosh** *(Cimicifuga racemosa)*, **Boneset** *(Eupatorium perfoliatum)*, **Bugleweed** *(Lycopus virginicus, L. americanus, L. europaeus)*, **Charcoal, Echinacea** *(Echinacea purpurea)*, **Garlic** *(Allium Sativum)*, **Ginger** *(Zingibar officinale)*, **Goldenseal** *(Hydrastis Canadensis)*, **Grapefruit Juice, Grapefruit Seed Extract, Gum Myrrh** *(Commiphora molmol)*, **Lady Slipper** *(Cypripedium calceolus)*, **Lobelia** *(Lobelia inflata)*, **Olive Leaf Extract** *(Olea europaea)*, **Pleurisy Root** *(Asclepias tuberose)*, **Red Clover** *(Trifolium pratense)*, **Raspberry Leaf** *(Rubus idaeus)*, **Skullcap** *(Scutellaria lateriflora)*, **Skunk Cabbage** *(Symplorcarpus foetidus)*, **Thyme (***Thymus vulgaris)*, **White Oak Bark** *(Quercus alba)*, **Wild Cherry Bark** *(Prunus serotina)*, **Wild Indigo** *(Baptisia Tinctoria)*, **Yarrow** *(Achillea milleforium)*

FORM: Capsules, teas, and tablets

HERBAL PROPHYLAXIS AND TREATMENT:

Prevention: Insure that a strict and sanitary hygiene is maintained. Use **antimicrobial herbs:** Take one capsule three times a day, three times a week (every other day) or one cup of tea made from any three-herb mixture, three times a week (every other day) for one to two weeks prior to traveling in an endemic typhoid area or during an outbreak.

Treatment: Drink copious amounts of various fluids daily for their rehydration effect throughout the course of the illness and convalescence. Use **antimicrobial herbs** and other **herbs** recommended in treatment instructions below: Take two to three capsules three times a day or one cup of tea made from any three-herb mixture three times a day for one week, then rotate combination of herbs each week until symptoms are gone.

- Get plenty of outdoor exercise and stay outdoors as much as possible.
- Drink lots of water.
- Help patient get plenty of rest and stay moderately warm.
- All patients with typhoid fever should have raw **garlic** to eat. It promotes circulation and kills the typhoid germ.
- Fruit juices and vegetable broths are important for recovery. Orange juice and oatmeal water taken at separate intervals are good nourishment.
- Induce profuse perspiration by the use of hot **yarrow** or **raspberry leaf** tea and by soaking in a tub of hot water with up to a pound of **ginger** and a teaspoon each of **mustard** and **cayenne** (*only experienced hydrotherapists should use this method*). With fevers, use moist heat to facilitate cleansing and eliminate the toxic backlog in the system, followed by a wet sheet treatment. (See Notes on Hydrotherapy in the Appendix.)
- Drink sufficient hot **echinacea** tea to induce diaphoresis, then administer hourly thereafter until the system is relieved of stagnated waste. It will also increase the patient's defense against infections and stimulate the process of detoxification of the liver and kidneys.
- Use compound antiseptic oil made from **oil of thyme, eugenol, menthol, eucalyptol,** and **olive oil** for the skin. May be taken internally or used externally with beneficial results. For use internally: use one teaspoon in one cup of water, sweetened with one tablespoon of honey, three to four times daily.
- For congestion with nerve irritation and delirium, combine **lady slipper** with **ginger** in a tea and give frequently.
- Give **pleurisy root** tea when the skin is dry and hot. Give **wild cherry bark** tea when there is diarrhea.
- Antispasmodic tincture using **lobelia, skullcap, skunk cabbage, gum myrrh,** and **black cohosh** may be very soothing. Give one teaspoon of antispasmodic tincture in a little warm water every half hour. Wash the body daily. Change bedclothes and sheets daily and give the patient warm water every two hours (with the juice of two to three lemons in a quart; give three to four cups each day).
- Give a daily high enema.
- The following antimicrobial herbs may be used: **aloe, buchu, calendula, Chinese skullcap, cloves, echinacea, elderberry, eucalyptus, garlic, ginseng, goldenseal, grapefruit seed extract, Japanese**

honeysuckle, lemon balm, lemon juice, licorice, lomatium root, myrrh, olive leaf, osha root, peppermint, rosemary, sage, tea tree, thyme, mint family of herbs.

- **Bugleweed** and **boneset** have been used frequently to reduce the high temperatures of typhoid fever without apparently weakening the patient.

CONTRAINDICATIONS: None

VARICELLA (CHICKENPOX)

Varicella–zoster virus (VZV) is known to cause two diseases: chickenpox (*varicella*) and shingles (*herpes zoster*). Chickenpox is a common contagious disease of children that usually has a benign course. The disease is spread by direct contact with infected lesions (pox) and by airborne droplets. It is communicable from one to two days before the rash develops until all the blister-like lesions have crusted, which takes an average of five or six days. It is one of the most infectious diseases. Chickenpox in adults or people with weakened immune systems can have serious complications. Second attacks of chickenpox are very rare. Shingles is caused by a reactivation of latent VZV. In other words, the virus lies dormant in nerve cells in the spine and can re-emerge in the form of shingles years after you have had chickenpox.

The typical rash of chickenpox is made up of groups of small, itchy blisters surrounded by inflamed skin. The rash usually begins as one or two lesions, quickly spreading throughout the body to include the trunk, scalp, face, arms, and legs. The total number of blisters varies greatly from person to person. Over four days, each blister tends to dry out and form a scab, which then falls off between nine and 13 days later. The rash is often preceded by a low-grade fever, fatigue, headache, and flu-like symptoms.

Chickenpox mainly occurs between two and eight years of age; it is much more severe if contracted as an adult. If a pregnant mother has it in the first four months of pregnancy, birth defects are possible. Once you have had it, you generally have lifetime immunity. This is one reason why the chickenpox vaccines are dangerous. It is better to get the disease as a child.

HERBALS AND BOTANICALS: **Aloe** *(Aloe vera/Aloe barbadensis/ Aloe ferox)*, **Black Walnut** *(Juglaris nigra)*, **Burdock Root** *(Arctium lappa)*, **Echinacea** *(Echinacea purpurea)*, **Garlic** *(Allium sativum)*, **Goldenseal** *(Hydrastis canadensis)*, **Lemon Balm** *(Melissa officinalis)*, **Licorice Root**

(*Glycyrrhiza glabra*), **Madonna Lily** (*Lilium candidum*), **Olive** (*Olea europaea*), **Rosehips** (*Rosa canina*), **White Willow** (*Salix alba, S. purpurea, S. fragilis*), **Yarrow** (*Achillea milleforium*)

FORM: Capsules, teas, and tablets

HERBAL PROPHYLAXIS AND TREATMENT:

Prevention: Chickenpox is transmitted by contact and by airborne droplets. Insure that a strict and sanitary hygiene is maintained. Use **antimicrobial herbs** and **other herbals:** Take one capsule three times a day, three times a week (every other day) or one cup of tea made from any three-herb mixture, three times a week (every other day) for one to two weeks prior to traveling in an endemic chickenpox area or during an outbreak.

Treatment: Drink copious amounts of various fluids daily for their rehydration effect throughout the course of the illness and convalescence. Use **antimicrobial herbs** and other **herbs** recommended in treatment instructions below: Take two to three capsules three times a day or one cup of tea made from any three-herb mixture three times a day for one week, then rotate combination of herbs each week until symptoms are gone.

- There is no evidence that antibiotics or corticosteroids are useful, and they should not be used.
- Itching may be relieved with applications of **calamine lotion**, moist **baking soda**, **honey**, or **starch** baths. Nails should be kept short and clean to minimize the possibility of infection from scratching. Scratching in young children may be discouraged by having them wear mittens or gloves, especially at night. Apply pressure to the area instead of scratching.
- **Tea tree oil** and **plantain** may also be used to soothe skin.
- **Catnip** tea with a little **molasses** is good during the fever. If the child is over age two, catnip tea enemas will help reduce the fever.
- **Licorice, echinacea,** and **aloe** may be used with good effect in addressing the virus that causes chickenpox. Also, the following antimicrobials may be used throughout the course of this disease: **buchu, calendula, Chinese skullcap, cloves, elderberry, eucalyptus, garlic, ginseng, goldenseal, grapefruit seed extract, Japanese honeysuckle, lemon balm, lemon juice, lomatium root, myrrh, olive leaf, osha root, peppermint, rosemary, sage, tea tree, thyme, mint family of herbs.**

- Aspirin should not be used to lower the fever, as about 10 percent of cases of Reyes Syndrome occur following chickenpox. Reyes Syndrome is a catastrophic disease in children, often causing death or an irreversible coma. Skincare for chickenpox includes a daily tepid bath and a daily change of clothes and linens. It is important to protect against chilling while bathing and at all other times, as chickenpox pneumonia can develop following exposure even in the convalescent stage.

- **Oatmeal** baths may be soothing. For an oatmeal bath, put one pound of uncooked oatmeal (or one heaping cup of uncooked rolled oats ground fine in a blender) into a bag made of two thicknesses of some material such as old sheeting or gauze. Float the bag in the bath water or hang it from the faucet and let the water entering the tub run through it. Use hot water first to soften the oatmeal. The bag may be used to gently sponge the body. Pat dry rather than rubbing dry after the bath.

- Saline rinses and gargles may be soothing to mouth lesions. Saline soaks (one level teaspoon salt to two cups of water) may be used for perineal lesions.

- At the onset of the disease, a deep, warm, 15-minute bath will encourage the pox to come out rapidly. Keep the water warm but not hot.

- Avoid constipation at all times.

- If you contract chickenpox as an adult, go on a fasting program of fresh fruits and vegetable juices, interspersed with light meals consisting of mashed bananas and raw applesauce. Insure that diet is fat-free and sugar-free.

- Isolation: Keep the infected child away from newborn infants, elderly people, and pregnant women who may not be immune to chickenpox. Do not send the child back to school until all the lesions have finished becoming crusted.

CONTRAINDICATIONS: None

WHOOPING COUGH (PERTUSSIS)

Pertussis is an infection of the breathing tract that is caused by a bacterium (*Bordetella pertussis*). It is also called whooping cough and is the "P" in the DTaP vaccine for children. It is an infectious disease, usually occurring in children, which begins with symptoms of a common cold but after about a week progresses to a violent, convulsive cough, often followed by vomiting. The cough mainly occurs at night, but as the illness progresses, it may appear during the day as well.

During a bout of coughing, you may hear the characteristic "whoop" as the child struggles to inhale. The child may cough as much as a dozen times with each breath, and the face may become blue. Whooping cough can be an exhausting and distressing experience for the parent and the child. Professional advice should be sought to treat whooping cough, especially in babies, and steps should be taken to avoid developing pneumonia or any damage to the lungs.

The vaccine against whooping cough is one of the most controversial of all immunizations. Cases of damaging side effects are well documented, including skin conditions and convulsions leading to permanent brain damage or, in more rare cases, death. There are also serious doubts about the effectiveness of the inoculation. When immunization was abandoned in Sweden and Germany due to concern about the potential side effects, absolutely no increase in whooping cough cases occurred. In the United States the immunization is still given routinely to infants as part of the DTaP or older DPT vaccine. *Many consider the pertussis vaccine to be the most dangerous of all shots.*[80]

HERBALS AND BOTANICALS: Anise Seed *(Pimpinella anisum)*, **Astragalus** *(Astragalus membraneceus)*, **Bayberry Bark** *(Myruca cerufera)*, **Catnip** *(Nepeta cateria)*, **Chamomile** *(Matricaria recutita)*, **Chestnut Leaves** *(Castanea sitvia)*, **Coltsfoot** *(Tussilago farfara)*, **Cramp Bark** *(Viburnum opulus)*, **Elecampane** *(Inula helenium)*, **Garlic** *(Allium sativum)*, **Hyssop** *(Hyssopus officinalis)*, **Licorice** *(Glycyrrhiza glabra)*, **Lobelia** *(Lobelia inflata)*, **Marshmallow Root** *(Althaea officinalis)*, **Mullein** *(Verbascum densiflorum)*, **Onion** *(Allium cepa)*, **Poke** *(Phytolacca americana L.)*, **Thyme** *(Thymus vulgaris)*, **Valerian** *(Valeriana officinalis)*, **Wild Cherry Bark** *(Prunus serotina)*, **Wild Lettuce** *(Lactuca virosa L.)*

FORM: Capsules, teas, and tablets

HERBAL PROPHYLAXIS AND TREATMENT:
Prevention: Insure that a strict and sanitary hygiene is maintained. Whooping cough occurs more frequently, and seriously, in overcrowded and unhygienic conditions and in cold weather. To prevent secondary infections use the following **antimicrobial herbs: anise, caraway, ginger, lemongrass, onion, wormwood, aloe,** and others listed in treatment section below: Take one capsule three times a day, three times a week (every other day) or one cup of tea made from any three-herb mixture, three

times a week (every other day) for one to two weeks prior to traveling in an endemic pertussis area or during an outbreak.

Treatment: The main objective in pertussis is to treat the cough. If this is done, the more serious phase can be aborted. Treatment should be done throughout the course of the illness and convalescence. Take **antitoxin herbs (goldenseal, gentian, bayberry, lemongrass)** and **antimicrobial herbs**: Take two to three capsules three times a day or one cup of tea made from any three-herb mixture three times a day for one week, then rotate combination of herbs each week until symptoms are gone.

- The following botanicals may be used for their antimicrobial properties: **anise, caraway, echinacea, garlic, ginger, goldenseal, grapefruit seed extract, lemongrass, licorice root, onion, thyme, wormwood.** **Echinacea** has particularly effective intestinal antiseptic properties. The following antimicrobials may be used with good effect: **aloe, buchu, calendula, Chinese skullcap, cloves, echinacea, elderberry, eucalyptus, garlic, ginseng, goldenseal, grapefruit seed extract, Japanese honeysuckle, lemon balm, lemon juice, licorice, lomatium root, myrrh, olive leaf, osha root, peppermint, rosemary, sage, tea tree, thyme, mint family of herbs.**
- Treat the cough! If you do so, the whooping cough phase can be entirely prevented. (Cough medicines, sedatives, expectorants, and antispasmodic drugs are useless.)
- In all kinds of coughs, first cleanse the system with high enemas and an herbal laxative (**senna** or **cascara segrada**).
- When cough is severe, have patient drink warm water, one cup after another, then stick your finger down his throat and have him vomit.
- The following teas are excellent for coughs: **wild cherry bark, black cohosh, flaxseed, rosemary, comfrey, horehound, hyssop, myrrh, white pine, bloodroot, red sage, blue violet, ginseng,** and **coltsfoot.** Prepare a tea and give every hour until the cough is better.
- Thick **slippery elm** tea is very good for whooping cough. Mix in a little lemon juice and drink it freely.
- **Thyme** and **echinacea** are very healing and have antiseptic action. They are especially beneficial for respiratory problems, and they have a soothing sedative action on the nerves. They help eliminate infections and restore health to children who are debilitated and exhausted by whooping cough.
- **Onion, raspberry leaves,** and **red clover** may be used as an antispasmodic tea.

- To help patient sleep at night (or any time), give patient a tepid bath (99° F.) for 10 to 15 minutes, with the head or face kept cool with an ice pack or wet washcloth.
- **Garlic** juice has remarkable penetrating power. The expressed juice of fresh garlic mixed with olive oil and rubbed on the chest, throat, and between the shoulder blades gives great relief in whooping cough.
- As soon as it is perceived that the problem is whooping cough, place patient on a full fruit-juice fast. First, give citrus juices. This can be followed by other fruit juices, then carrots and other vegetable juices, and then clear vegetable broth. Vitamins A and C in large doses can be given with juices.
- To cut the phlegm, use **bayberry** tea as a gargle (swallow after gargling). Crushed **garlic** with **honey** can help to clear the throat.
- Do not overeat during whooping cough; it prolongs the disease and leads to complications. If it is a breastfed infant, do not overfeed either. The child may be thirsty, not hungry.
- It is good to soak the feet in hot water, with a little mustard and salt added to water.
- A little petroleum jelly can be placed under the child's nose and around the lips to prevent skin irritation.
- As soon as the child finishes vomiting, rinse his mouth to get rid of the hydrochloric acid, which could damage his teeth.
- Warm vapor inhalations are often very helpful. They can be given every two to four hours, according to the severity of the case. Place a humidifier or carefully guarded steam kettle on a hot plate in patient's room.
- Keep patient's room well-ventilated day and night, but avoid drafts.
- If the weather is warm, sunny, and not too damp or dusty, keep patient outdoors most of the day. But patient should not overexert himself in play or become chilled.
- When there is sunshine, have the patient sunbathe in fresh air each day.
- Keep affected child isolated from other children.
- Do not give aspirin to a child or youth with a fever. It could lead to Reyes Syndrome and possibly to death.
- During the catarrhal stage (when mucous membranes of the head and neck are inflamed and dry coughing may occur): Choose four herbs from the above lists. Combine in equal parts in a tea (one-half cup every three to four hours), a tincture, or glycerite (30 drops every three to four hours).

- During the paroxysmal stage (when the onset of coughing or other symptoms is sudden and severe): In addition to the above formula, combine two parts of **catnip** with two to four of the other **antispasmodic herbs** in a tincture or glycerite (20 drops every one to two hours).

- Immune-stimulating herbs **(coneflower, echinacea, garlic, astragalus,** or other immune-enhancing herbs from chapter 5) may also be used.

CONTRAINDICATIONS: None

YELLOW FEVER

Yellow fever is a viral disease endemic to tropical and subtropical Africa and America, with epidemics occurring elsewhere on occasion. It is transmitted by the bites of *Aedes aegypti* mosquitoes or those of several close relatives.

The incubation period is three to six days. Many mild cases of yellow fever occur, with only a small percentage developing a severe form of the disease. Symptoms include fever, chills, aching muscles, headache, possibly flushed and swollen face, bloodshot eyes, vomiting, and pain in the upper abdomen. Most cases clear up at this stage. In severe cases the onset is more violent, and jaundice and hemorrhages develop by about the fourth day. Severe cases can be fatal, with mortality rates varying from 7 to 50 percent.

The inoculation is considered to be over 90 percent effective; however, it does affect the immune system detrimentally and is contraindicated for people taking steroids and those with a history of allergies, cancer, or positive HIV status. Usually the immunization is also advised against for pregnant women and infants. An international certificate of vaccination against yellow fever is required when entering some countries. Taking precautions to avoid being bitten by mosquitoes is essential in preventing the disease.

HERBALS AND BOTANICALS: African Marigold *(Targetes erecta),* **Aloe Vera** *(aloe spp.),* **Blessed Thistle** *(Cnicus benedictus),* **Catnip** *(Nepeta cataria),* **Devil's Claw** *(Harpagiphytum procumbens),* **Lemongrass** *(Cymbopigin citrates),* **Licorice** *(Glycyrrhiza glabra),* **Lobelia** *(Lobelia inflata),* **Milk Thistle** *(Silybum marianum),* **Schisandra** *(Schisandra chinensis),* **St. John's Wort** *(Hypericum perforatum),* **White Willow Bark** *(Salix alba, S. cinereas)*

FORM: Capsules, teas, and tablets

HERBAL PROPHYLAXIS AND TREATMENT:

Prevention: Use **mosquito-repellent** or **aromatic herbs (African marigold** or *Tagetes erecta, tageta minuta,* **lemongrass,** *Artemisia annua,* **garlic) and anti-mosquito** and **antimicrobial herbs (Artemisia** or **Sweet Annie, astragalus, black adler bark, cinchona bark, echinacea, garlic, goldenseal, gentian root, licorice, milk thistle, neem tree, quassia bark, white willow bark):** Take one capsule three times a day, three times a week (every other day) or one cup of tea made from any three-herb mixture, three times a week (every other day) for one to two weeks prior to traveling in an endemic area (infected with *Aedes aegypti* or closely related mosquito) or during an outbreak.

- The best protection from yellow fever is to prevent mosquito bites. Control mosquito breeding environment; use screens and nets impregnated with repellants and insecticides over bed.
- Mosquito repellents: Use aromatic herbs inside the house: **African marigold** or *Tagetes erecta, tageta minuta,* **lemongrass,** *Artemisia annua.*
- Use 8 to 10 drops of **Grapefruit Seed Extract (GSE)** three times a day or tablets equal to 10 to 15 drops of GSE for prevention.
- Eating one or two cloves of raw garlic each day will discourage mosquitoes from landing on skin.
- **Catnip** has been used as a mosquito repellant in many cultures.

Treatment: Continue to use mosquito-repellent or aromatic herbs listed above in Prevention section. Drink copious amounts of various fluids daily for their rehydration effect throughout the course of the illness and convalescence. Use **antitoxin herbs (goldenseal, gentian, bayberry, lemongrass):** Take two to three capsules three times a day or one cup of tea made from any three-herb mixture three times a day for one week, then rotate combination of herbs each week until symptoms are gone.

- Antibiotics do not have any significant beneficial effect on yellow fever virus and should not be used.
- The following antimicrobials may be used throughout the course of this disease: **aloe, buchu, calendula, Chinese skullcap, cloves, echinacea, elderberry, eucalyptus, garlic, ginseng, goldenseal, grapefruit seed extract, Japanese honeysuckle, lemon balm, lemon juice, licorice, lomatium root, myrrh, olive leaf, osha root, peppermint, rosemary, sage, tea tree, thyme, mint family of herbs.**

- **Blessed thistle, St. John's wort, licorice, schisandra** may be used as antivirals and to protect the liver.
- Maintain a vegetarian diet rich in vegetables and fresh fruits, especially those high in vitamin C, such as lemons, bitter oranges, kiwis, pineapples, mangos, and papayas.
- Drink plenty of fluids, water, natural juices, potassium-rich broths, and vegetable broth. These should be cool, not cold.
- **Charcoal** poultices may be helpful for painful joints and enlarged liver and spleen.
- A well-timed hydrotherapy treatment can benefit all yellow fever patients. The treatment should be timed to the cycles of fever, since the temperature will usually go up at the same time each day and in the same cycle (such as every four hours). General revulsive fomentation over the liver and spleen with two minutes of cold mitten friction should be used. A hot and cold contrast shower at the beginning of symptoms may reduce symptoms. The shower should be three minutes of hot followed by 30 seconds of cold for four changes. Have the patient rest for at least 30 minutes following treatment. Note: If daily chills begin, note the time of day and take a hot and cold shower or steam treatment 30 minutes before onset on subsequent days.
- For high fevers (above 104° F.) mild hydrotherapy may reduce the temperature. A wet sheet pack with a cool cloth to the head will alleviate chills when applied for 20 minutes. A cool water enema may also bring the temperature down. Be sure to keep patient well hydrated with **catnip** tea.
- Give an emetic to induce vomiting if there is a lot of phlegm: **lobelia, peach leaves, ragwort, white willow, myrica,** and **bayberry bark.**
- **Grapefruit, lemon,** and **ginger** may be used as a diaphoretic.

CONTRAINDICATIONS: None

APPENDIX

Notes on Hydrotherapy

Hydrotherapy, or water therapy, is the skillful use of water (hot, cold, steam, or ice) to relieve discomfort, boost the immune system and promote physical well-being. There are many different types of therapeutic treatments ranging from a hot foot bath to a general revulsive to the chest to a contrast shower.

Hydrotherapy can affect all the systems of the body: respiratory, circulatory, endocrine, cardiovascular, the immune system, and so on. For example, a hot and cold contrast shower has the unique ability to boost the immune system by increasing the quantity and proficiency of white blood cells (T-cells). *It is customary to pray before each hydrotherapy treatment, inviting the Great Physician's participation. This improves the patient's confidence.*

In order to become thoroughly proficient in hydrotherapy and its benefits, refer to a textbook on the topic. A text that I find to be helpful is found in the Suggested Reading section of this Appendix.

Common Hydrotherapy Treatments

Compresses

Both hot and cold compresses actually start off as cold compresses. A cloth is dipped in ice-cold water and left on the affected part of the body for a certain period of time. In the case of a cold compress, the pack is replaced by an equally cold pack once it begins to lose its chill. In the case of a hot compress, the pack is left on and allowed to heat up by the warmth of the body. Both types of compresses are used in various ways, especially to treat acute injuries.

Cold Compress

A cold compress is a local application of cold given by means of a cloth wrung from cold water. Either hand towels or cotton cloth may be used. This treatment is helpful for fever, pain due to edema or trauma, congestion of sinuses, and congestive headaches.

- Use Turkish towels to protect the bedding, as well as patient's clothing, from becoming wet.
- Fold two or three towels (or cloths) to a desired size, then dip them into cold water and wring them out—but only enough to prevent dripping. (Better: take the wet cloths out of a container of ice cubes

and quickly apply them. In this way the compresses will be far colder.)

- Lay cloths on the afflicted part.
- Replace the compress with a fresh cold one every one to five minutes. A set of two compresses will be needed so that they can be continually alternated. The thicker the compress, the less often will it have to be replaced with a new one.
- Cold compresses can be placed on the head, neck, over the heart or lungs, on the abdomen, spine, and so on. When applied to the head, they need to be pressed down firmly, especially over the forehead and the temporal arteries (these arteries are to the right and left of the forehead, just above and to the front of the ears).

Contrast Bath
The contrast bath consists of immersing a body part alternately in hot and cold water. (The hot and cold water may be applied with a wash cloth to body areas that cannot be easily immersed in water.)

- Begin with a hot bath. Start with milder heat; increase the heat as tolerated. After three or four minutes (or time specified for treatment) transfer to the cold water bath for 30 to 60 seconds.
- During the treatment, keep the hot and cold baths at the desired temperature by adding hot or cold water as needed.
- Place a cold compress to the head if sweating occurs.
-
- Make five to seven changes per treatment. Treat one to four times per day.
- After the last change, thoroughly dry the treated body part.
- If sweating occurs, dry the entire body, remove damp clothing, and dress in clean, dry garments.

Gargle
Gargling is a great way to kill bacteria in your mouth and throat area.

- Pour the gargle solution into a clean glass or paper cup. If you pour it into the lid of the container being used, you risk contaminating the solution.
- If you gargle with salt water, dissolve one-half teaspoon salt in 8 ounces of warm water.
- Slide the solution quickly over the tongue.

- Throw the head back and stop the solution right before it reaches the epiglottis (the cartilaginous flap in the back of the throat). You will know the solution is resting on the right spot if you sense the need to gag or swallow.
- Make the solution bubble and gurgle for at least 45 seconds. Pull your tongue back a little and blow air through your throat slowly. Be sure to keep your head way back and remember to keep the solution right in front of the epiglottis. That is where the germs are concentrated, far back and out of sight. Try not to swallow any of the solution.
- Drop your head down and spit the solution out.
- Repeat several times.

Contrast Shower

This is an abrupt, alternating shower, changing back and forth from hot to cold. It is a vigorous tonic and stimulant for the body.

- Begin with the hot water at a temperature of 106-110° F., then quickly raise the temperature to the upper limit of tolerance. Hold it there for two minutes.
- Turn the valves quickly to full cold. Hold it there for 30 seconds.
- Reverse again to hot for about two minutes, then back to cold for 30 seconds again.
- Do three complete cycles of hot and cold, finishing with the cold water.
- Dry well with sheet and towel. Rest for 10 to 15 minutes after the treatment.

Fomentation

A fomentation consists of a local application of moist heat to the surface of the body to affect a specific internal organ (such as liver or spleen). It is used as an analgesic for pain, to increase blood flow peripherally in order to relieve congestion internally, and for stimulation and sedation. A hot foot bath may be done simultaneously. (A **general revulsive fomentation** consists of treatment focused on the lung area.)

- Place a dry towel on top of the body part being treated before putting the heated moist fomentation on the patient. Then cover the fomentation with another dry towel.
- If the fomentation becomes too hot, lift it off the skin and put another dry towel under the fomentation.

- Leave the fomentation in place for the specified length of time or until the fomentation cools.
- Remove the cooled fomentation and briskly rub the heated area with a cold washcloth for approximately one minute. Thoroughly dry the treated area before applying the next fomentation. Remember to keep the patient completely covered at all times during the treatment.
- Place the second fomentation on the treated area and repeat the steps until the treatment is completed. A treatment consists of three to five fomentation applications. As soon as the patient begins to sweat, put cool washcloths on the head and neck.
- During the treatment, have the patient drink water frequently to replace fluid lost from sweating.
- Keep the feet warm by periodically adding hot water to a foot bath. Place your hand between the hot water being poured and the patient's feet (to avoid burning the feet).
- After removing the last fomentation, briskly rub the treated area with a cold washcloth and then dry it.
- Lift the feet out of the hot water bath and point the toes upward. Quickly pour cold water over the feet.
- Thoroughly dry feet and toes, then place warm socks or slippers on the feet to avoid chilling.
- Remove sweat from remainder of the body by briskly rubbing the skin with cold wash cloths and drying it thoroughly. Replace damp clothing with clean, dry garments.
- Have patient rest in bed for approximately one hour.

Oatmeal Baths

An oatmeal bath is often used for soaking the body. It is soothing to the skin because of a starch-like substance and can be use for many skin conditions.

- Put one pound of uncooked oatmeal (or one heaping cup of uncooked rolled oats ground fine in a blender) into a bag made of two thicknesses of some material such as old sheeting or gauze.
- Float the bag in the bath water or hang it from the faucet and let the water entering the tub run through it.
- Use hot water first to soften the oatmeal.
- The bag may be used to gently sponge the body. Pat dry rather than rubbing dry after the bath.

Hot Foot Bath

The hot foot bath consists of placing the feet in hot water deep enough to completely cover the ankles. The hot foot bath affects the circulation of the entire body. Heat expands or dilates the blood vessels of the feet, which moves the blood from other areas to the feet. The increased blood flow to the feet relieves congestion of the blood in the brain, lungs, and abdominal organs.

- Place feet in a tub of hot water as hot as the patient can endure. Keep it hot for 20 to 30 minutes by adding more hot water as tolerated.
- Keep the head cool with a cloth wrung from ice water.
- At the conclusion of the hot foot bath, remove the feet from the tub and pour over them the ice water used to keep the head cool.
- Dress the patient warmly (particularly the feet), to prevent the slightest chilling of the skin in the extremities.

Enema, High Enema

Water is placed in the large bowel (the large intestine) in order to remove impacted wastes and toxic substances. Either an enema bag or colonic apparatus can be used for this purpose (follow the general instructions given with your apparatus). Different water temperatures (hot, warm, tepid, or cold) may be used in the procedure.

Sitz Bath

This bath is used to treat problems in the pelvic and genital areas. There are six types of sitz baths: cold, prolonged cold, neutral, very hot, revulsive, and the contrast (or alternating hot and cold) sitz bath. The water temperature determines the effect upon the body. The contrast or alternating sitz bath will be described here.

- Situate two tubs side by side; they should be large enough to submerge pelvic region. Two smaller tubs should be place in front of each tub for the feet.
- Fill one large tub with hot (106 to 115° F.) water and the other with cold (55 to 65° F.) water.
- Foot baths for both tubs should be 105 to 115° F.
- Pelvic region should be submerged in the hot water for three minutes, then alternate to cold water tub for 30 seconds for three or four changes, always ending in cold.
- During the procedure a cold compress should be applied to the head and neck.

- When the bath is complete, the patient should dry thoroughly and rest for approximately 30 minutes

Wet Sheet Pack

A wet sheet pack is a procedure in which the whole body is wrapped in a wet sheet, which in turn is wrapped in a dry blanket for regulating evaporation.

- The blanket should be spread on the bed with its edges hanging over the edge of the bed. The upper end should be about eight inches from the head of the bed. Then spread a linen sheet wrung out in cold water over the blanket so that its end is slightly below the upper end of the blanket.
- The patient should lie on the sheet with his shoulders about three inches below the upper edge. The wet sheet should be weakly wrapped around the body of the patient, drawn in, and tightly tucked between the legs and also between the body and the arms.
- The sheet should be folded over the shoulders and across the neck. Now the blanket should be drawn tightly around the body and tucked in along the side in a similar manner, pulling it tightly. The ends should be doubled up at the feet. Refer to a good book on hydrotherapy for detailed instructions and diagrams for folding the sheet and blanket.
- A turkish towel should be placed below the chin to protect the face and neck from coming into contact with the blanket and to exclude outside air more effectively.
- The head should be covered with a wet cloth so that the skull remains cold.
- The feet should be kept warm during the entire treatment. If the patient's feet are cold, place hot water bottles near them to hasten reaction. The pack is administered for 30 to 60 minutes until the patient begins to perspire profusely. He may be given cold or hot water to drink.

Poultice

This is a salve of one or more ingredients combined with a little hot water. It is then spread on a damp cloth and placed over an infection (generally but not always an infection which is on or just below the surface of the skin). Poultices are made of charcoal, flaxseed, clay, garlic, comfrey, hops, mustard, and so on.

- Assemble everything needed and prepare the poultice in a warm room.
- Place the salve on a damp cloth, then place that on the area to be treated. Cover with plastic and then with a wool cloth over that. Pin or tape the poultice in place. Leave it on overnight or as directed.
- When removing it, be careful not to spill used ingredients on the floor. Rub the treated area with ice or with a very cold, wet wash-cloth. You may wish to renew the poultice with fresh salve and clean cloths.

Travel Kit/First-Aid Kit

A natural-remedy travel kit/first-aid kit is a simple and practical collection of herbal agents to treat minor injuries safely and effectively at home or while traveling. Ideally, it should include a user-friendly first-aid booklet that provides explanations of the herbs and their uses in the care of cuts, burns, bruises, sore gums, and more.

Be sure to include dosage information on the bottles as well as in the instruction booklet, which can be nothing more than 3x5 cards that you cover with see-through packing tape to waterproof and keep clean.

Essential Oils

Citronella Oil
Citronella oil is a repellent that can be diluted and applied to the skin or burned in a room as a repellent. It is used against mosquitoes and other insects.

Garlic Oil
Antimicrobial and antimycotic. It may be used for high blood pressure, colds, coughs, whooping cough, earaches, gastrointestinal ailments, and bronchitis.

Lavender Oil
Antiseptic and anti-inflammatory. Pour onto minor burns and scalds or hold near the nose and inhale the vapors when feeling faint. Add a few drops to a bath for stress or insomnia. May be used in a bath or massaged onto the temple to relieve a tension headache.

Peppermint
A little on the temples can help you stay awake, and a few drops in water will settle an upset stomach.

Tea Tree Oil
Antiseptic and antiviral. Called a "first-aid kit in a bottle," tea tree (*Melaleuca leucadendron*) oil has strong antifungal and antimicrobial properties with antiseptic abilities. It can be used for chest and fungal infections (steam inhalation), pus-filled wounds or burns, cold/flu, cold sores, and herpes lesions. For use with earaches and on sensitive skin, dilute with equal parts olive oil. Use sparingly; tea tree oil goes a long way.

Eucalyptus Oil

Germicidal and antimicrobial. Maybe used for wound healing, abscesses, burns, ulcers, and insect bites or stings. It also suppresses coughs, loosens phlegm, and improves lung function. Eucalyptus oil is also great for use in a sickroom environment to kill germs in the air and reduce the number of airborne bacteria.

Herbal Extracts

Herbal tinctures and extracts are the preferred form of medicine, as they are assimilated quickly and administered easily. Tincturing also extracts valuable constituents not found in teas, since certain active plant properties are only soluble in alcohol. If you dislike the alcohol, you can reduce its presence somewhat by placing the drops in one-half cup of hot, boiled water and allowing it to sit for 15 minutes. You can also mix the extract with juice to disguise the taste. To keep things in perspective, it has been said that there's more alcohol in a ripe banana than in the suggested dosage of herbal extracts.

Cayenne

Five to 10 drops diluted in two ounces of water can be used externally (cayenne should only be used medicinally, not as a spice or condiment) for frostbite and hypothermia. It moves the blood from the center of the body to the peripheral areas, warming hands and feet. A couple of drops under the tongue will help to revive someone in shock or trauma. Used externally for heavily bleeding lacerations, it will coagulate the blood to stanch the flow (though it stings a bit).

Valerian

As an antispasmodic and painkiller, this herb relieves intestinal and menstrual cramps, headaches, and general aches or pains. As a nervine, it will bring sleep to an exhausted person. The dosage range is 30 to 60 drops.

Echinacea

Besides possessing the ability to increase the supply of white blood cells to an infected area, thus boosting the immune system, echinacea is also antibiotic and antibacterial to gram-positive bacteria such as strep or staph. It's helpful with fevers, poisoning, or any type of internal infection and has reportedly been used for poisonous insect and snake bites by native Plains tribes. Echinacea is a good preventative and supportive herb for the onset of the flu or common cold. The dosage ranges from 30 to 60 drops, with the higher ranges used for fevers and acute situations. For toothaches, it can be massaged into the surrounding gums and teeth. For poisonous bites, 60 drops every 15 minutes is appropriate.

Milk Thistle Combination
This can include milk thistle, burdock, and kelp in equal parts. This herb acts to leach heavy metals and radiation toxicity from the thyroid, blood, and liver, and it also protects the liver against further damage. Good to take before and after dental x-rays and after taking Tylenol or Advil.

Quassia
An antimicrobial, this herb is traditionally used for bacterial diarrhea, dysentery, and giardia—a lower gastrointestinal complaint contracted by drinking contaminated water. It may be used to treat suspected bad water.

Lobelia, Bayberry Bark, Peach Leaves, Pokeweed
These are standard remedies to promote vomiting and should only be used in certain types of poisoning.

Powdered Herbs

Slippery Elm Capsules
Used for food poisoning, this powder combines with and buffers poisons in the stomach and bowels to decrease toxic absorption. It can soothe mucous membranes and settle an upset stomach.

Ginger Root Capsules
Use two caps for motion and morning sickness. It's also effective for nausea caused by flu or bad food.

Marshmallow-Peppermint Oil Capsules
This is an easy-to-make combination of four parts marshmallow powder to one part peppermint oil. The powder in this formula is basically a vehicle for the peppermint oil to reach the small intestines without dissolving in the stomach. The capsules reduce intestinal cramping that can accompany any gastrointestinal tract infection. For children not able to swallow capsules, you can dissolve the contents in four cups of juice or sweetened water.

Poultice Combination Powder
This should consist of at least one antibacterial herb, one antifungal, an emollient, and an astringent. A possible combination can contain equal parts gentian, myrrh gum, goldenseal, and marshmallow. This powder can be stored in a plastic zipper bag and makes a nice dust for sore feet, lacerations (it will stop excess bleeding), diaper rash, infections, insect bites, or inflamed eyes (it is cooling and soothing). A tea of these herbs can be used externally as a wash. For foreign objects in the eye, make a paste by adding water to the mix and bandage it over the closed eyelid to draw the object out and soothe the eye simultaneously.

Charcoal
Charcoal is a simple remedy that should be in every home. It is formed from charred wood when wood is heated in the absence of air. Charcoal has the unique ability to *adsorb,* or remove, poisonous gases, drugs, toxic chemicals, infectious bacteria, and viruses. It can be used internally as a capsule, a powder, or in tablet form for poisoning, nausea and vomiting, diarrhea, intestinal gas, sore throat, and bad breath. Externally, it may be used with or without flaxseed as a poultice or included in a bath for insect bites and stings, spider bites and snake bites, skin lesions from poisonous plants, skin infections, and as a deodorizing agent.

Salves

A good all-purpose salve is essential. You want one that will draw and shrink swollen tissues, fight bacteria, and soothe compromised tissues. Here is a list of common herbs that may be used in salves:

Emollients
Marshmallow, slippery elm, plantain, comfrey, and mullein.

Antimicrobials
Echinacea, goldenseal, yerba mansa, Oregon grape, osha, propolis, myrrh gum, garlic, calendula, chamomile, chaparral, gentian, and usnea.

Astringents
Horsetail, bistort, geranium, rose, alum, yarrow, witch hazel, yellow dock, and St. John's wort.

Altitude Sickness
Gingko biloba, cloves, garlic, gingko, horse balm, and the mint family of herbal agents.

Notes to Travelers

Take some basic steps to help yourself stay healthy when traveling.

Preparation:

Research the areas you will be visiting, consult the relevant disease and alternative vaccine sections of this book, and take the appropriate remedies you will need. The Centers for Disease Control (CDC), your local health department, and your travel/tour service will be able to provide more detail regarding your travel plans.

One should start on an immune-enhancing diet before a trip. It is possible to have a healthy vacation abroad if you take some basic precautions.

What to consider taking with you:
- A basic travel/first-aid kit (see earlier section in Appendix)
- Altitude sickness herbs (gingko biloba, cloves, garlic, horse balm, mint family of herbs)
- A supply of sterile dressing
- A one-cup size electric element for boiling water to drink and brush teeth (available at camping supply stores)
- Insect repellent (such as citronella essential oil)
- Mosquito net

What to avoid:
- Avoid drinking or cleaning your teeth in contaminated water. (This includes avoiding ice. Moreover, travelers must not assume incorrectly that food and water onboard a commercial aircraft are safe.)
- Avoid eating doubtful foods, such as meat, salad, and melons.
- Avoid swimming in contaminated water.
- Take precautions to avoid insect bites.

Travel Vaccines—Two Categories:

Recommended vaccinations:

Travelers are advised by the CDC and other travel service organizations to take certain recommended vaccines based upon the illnesses found in their country of destination. These recommendations depend on a number of factors included in your itinerary, such as whether you will be spending time in rural areas, the season of the year, your age, and your health status.

Required vaccination:
The only vaccination required by International Health Regulation is the yellow fever vaccination for travel to certain countries in sub-Saharan Africa and tropical South America. Meningococcal vaccination is required by the government of Saudi Arabia for annual travel during the Hajj. Some countries do not require an International Certificate of Vaccination (ICV) for infants younger than 6 months of age.

Waiver Letters from Physicians:
A physician's letter clearly stating contraindications to vaccination is acceptable to some governments. Ideally, it should be written on letter-head stationary and bear the stamp used by the health department and official immunization centers to validate the ICV. Travelers should be advised that issuance of a waiver does not guarantee that the destination country will accept it. Immunization recommendations for international travel can be obtained from the Centers for Disease Control (CDC).

Note to Missionaries

Missionaries should take the same precautions any traveler would take to stay healthy while traveling and living in their assigned area. After the appropriate research, consult the relevant disease and alternative vaccine sections of this book and make preparations for your extended stay. Remember, as a missionary you will have to make long-term plans to be safe and healthy during your visit.

Notes to Parents

Many healthcare professionals will put pressure on you to vaccinate your child starting soon after birth. If you have chosen not to do so, then be prepared with some facts before appointments with doctors, social workers, and so on. There is no legal requirement for you to have your child vaccinated in the United States and many other countries.

If you have not made up your mind about immunization, then join a support group and talk to other parents who believe as you believe. Also, look at the websites suggested in this section and consider talking to a natural-remedies healthcare professional.

As with so many issues that come up for a parent, making decisions on behalf of someone else can seem very difficult. It is even more difficult if you are considering going against established dogmas and orthodox opinions. Remember, you're not alone. Many parents are choosing to maintain their family's immunity with lifestyle and herbal methods.

It is also advisable to do the following:

Make contact with a practitioner you can trust before your child becomes ill.

Keep a stock of basic remedies in the house and in your first-aid kit / travel kit. (See previous sections of Appendix.)

Exemptions

Your Right to Accept or Refuse Vaccinations
The question "Can I refuse a vaccine?" is being asked more and more by parents, travelers, and missionaries as they hear and read about the association between vaccines and serious health conditions. Although there are no federal mandates that force parents to have their children vaccinated, state laws essentially act as such. Many parents are unaware that they can get an exemption from vaccinating their child based on medical, philosophical, or religious reasons, depending on the laws of their particular state. Your state's public health department, the public library, and other agencies will provide you with the needed information.

If a child goes to school without meeting state vaccination requirements, the child can be removed from school. There have also been instances where state officials have charged parents with neglect for failing to vaccinate children with all mandated vaccines. Therefore, parents need to have full access to information allowing them to weigh the risks and benefits of the many recommended vaccines.

Immigrants and missionaries to the United States may receive a waiver if requested upon entering the country. This request should occur as early in the process as possible or during the physical examination interview.

Legal Exemptions to Vaccinations
There are three major categories of vaccination exemptions available for those who believe the risk of injury is too great. These exemptions are medical, religious, and philosophical.

These exemptions are worded differently in each state. To use an exemption for yourself or your child, you must know specifically what the law says in your state. To obtain a copy of your laws, ask your local reference librarian to help you. You may also find updated information by searching the Internet.

Note: The following exemptions are current at the time of publication.

Philosophical Exemption: The following 18 states allow exemption to vaccination based on philosophical beliefs: Arizona, California, Colorado, Idaho, Louisiana, Maine, Michigan, Minnesota, New Mexico, North Dakota, Ohio, Oklahoma, Rhode Island, Texas, Utah, Vermont, Washington, and Wisconsin.

In many of these states, individuals must object to all vaccines, not just a particular vaccine, in order to use the philosophical objection or personal conviction exemption. Many state legislators are being urged by federal health officials and medical organizations to revoke this exemption to vaccination. If you are objecting to vaccination based on philosophical or personal conviction, keep an eye on your state legislature as public health officials seek to amend state laws to eliminate this exemption.

Religious Exemption: All states allow a religious exemption to vaccination except Mississippi and West Virginia.

The religious exemption is intended for people who possess a sincere religious belief against vaccination to the extent that if the state forced vaccination, it would be an infringement on their right to exercise their religious beliefs. Some state laws define religious exemptions broadly to include personal religious beliefs, similar to personal philosophical beliefs. Other states require an individual who claims a religious exemption to be a member of the First Church of Christ, Scientist (Christian Science) or another bona fide religion whose written tenets include prohibition of invasive medical procedures such as vaccination.

Some laws require a signed affidavit from the pastor of the church, while others allow the parent to sign a notarized waiver. Prior to registering your child for school, you must check your state law to verify what your health department requires to prove your religious beliefs. The religious exemption is granted based on the First Amendment of the Constitution, which is the right to freely exercise your religion.

Because citizens are protected under the First Amendment of the Constitution, a state must have a "compelling State interest" before this right can be taken away. One "compelling State interest" is the spread of communicable diseases. In state court cases which have set precedent on this issue, the freedom to act according to your own religious belief is subject to reasonable regulation, with the justification that it must not threaten the welfare of society as a whole. In this instance, parents can elect to homeschool their children.

Medical Exemption: All 50 states allow medical exemption to vaccination. Proof of medical exemption must take the form of a signed statement by a Medical Doctor (M.D.) or Doctor of Osteopathy (D.O.) saying that the administering of one or more vaccines would be detrimental to the health of the individual.

Most doctors follow the American Academy of Pediatrics (AAP) and Centers for Disease Control (CDC) guidelines. Most states do not allow

Doctors of Chiropractic (D.C.) to write medical exemptions to vaccination. Some states will accept a private physician's written exemption without question. Other states allow the state health department to review the doctor's exemption and revoke it if health department officials don't think the exemption is justified.

Proof of Immunity: Most states will allow exemption to vaccination for certain diseases if proof of immunity can be shown to exist. Immunity can be proven if you or your child have had the natural disease or have been vaccinated. You have to check your state laws to determine which vaccines in your state can be exempted if proof of immunity is demonstrated.

Private medical laboratories can take blood (a titer test) and analyze it to measure the level of antibodies, for example, to measles or pertussis, that are present in the blood. If the antibody level is high enough, according to accepted standards, you have obtained proof of immunity and may be able to use this for an exemption to vaccination.

References

[1] P. Smith, S. Chu, and L. Barker, "Children Who Have Received No Vaccines: Who Are They and Where Do They Live?" *Pediatrics*, vol. 114, No. 1 (July 2004), pp. 187-195.

[2] http://www/autism-society.org, http://www.dds.ca.gov, http://www.gti.net/truegrit, http://www.autism.com/ari

[3] *The Lancet*, 1 Dec. 1980, p. 73.

[4] National Vaccine Information Center, 2 March 1994.

[5] "Abstract," *Science*, 4 April 1977.

[6] *British Medical Journal* 283: 696-697, 1981.

[7] M. Burnet and D. White, *The Natural History of Infectious Disease* (Cambridge, 1972), p. 16.

[8] Strebel, et al, "Epidemiology in the U.S. One Decade After the Last Reported Case of Indigenous Wild Virus Associated Disease," *Clinical Infectious Diseases,* (Centers for Disease Control, Feb. 1992), pp. 568-79.

[9] *Physician's Desk Reference* (PDR), 50th ed., "Medical Economics" (1996), pp. 1388-1390.

[10] Ibid, pp. 885-886 and 891-892.

[11] J. Butel, et al, "Molecular Evidence of Simian Virus 40 Infections in Children," *The Journal of Infectious Diseases,* Sept. 1999, 180:884-887.

[12] PDR, 50th ed., pp. 872-875.

[13] Ibid.

[14] Ibid.

[15] Richard Moskowitz, M.D., "Immunizations: The Other Side," *Mothering,* Spring 1984, p. 34.

[16] *Immunization: Survey of Recent Research,* (United States Department of Health and Human Services, April 1983), p. 76.

[17] "Nature and Rates of Adverse Reactions Associated with DPT and DT Immunizations...," *Pediatrics*, vol. 68, no. 5 (Nov. 1981).

[18] Walene James, *Immunization: The Reality Behind the Myth* (South Hadley, MA: Bergin and Garvey, 1988), p. 14.

[19] W.C. Torch, "Diptheria-Pertussis-Tetanus (DPT) Immunization: A Potential Cause of Sudden Infant Death Syndrome (SIDS)" (Amer. Academy of Neurology, 34th Annual Meeting, Apr. 25 - May 1, 1982), *Neurology* 32(4), pt. 2.

[20] PDR, pp. 875-879 and 892-895.

[21] Ibid.

[22] Robert Mendelsohn, M.D., *How to Raise A Healthy Child In Spite of Your Doctor* (Chicago: Contemporary Books, 1984), p. 223.

[23] Ibid, pp. 244-246.

[24] Isaac Golden, Ph.D., Vaccination? *A Review of Risks and Alternatives* (Geelong, Victoria, Australia: Arum Healing Centre, 1991), p. 31.

[25] Richard Moskowitz, M.D., "Immunizations: The Other Side," *Mothering,* Spring 1984, p. 34.

[26] Isaac Golden, Ph.D., *Vaccination? A Review of Risks and Alternatives,* p. 71.

[27] R. Mendelsohn, *How to Raise a Healthy Child*, p. 217.

[28] John Frank, Jr., M.D., et al., "Measles Elimination: Final Impediments," 20th Immunization Conference Proceedings, May 6-9, 1985, p. 21.

[29] *Infectious Diseases* (Jan. 1982), p. 21.

[30] PDR, pp. 1610-1611.

[31] PDR, pp. 1687-1689.

[32] Sara Solovitch, "Do Vaccines Spur Autism in Kids?" *San Jose Mercury News*, 25 May 1999.

[33] PDR, pp. 1687-89 and 1610-1611.

[34] Richard Moskowitz, M.D., "Immunizations: The Other Side," *Mothering*, Spring 1984, p. 35.

[35] PDR, pp. 1708-1709.

[36] Ibid.

[37] R. Mendelsohn, *How to Raise a Healthy Child*, p. 218.

[38] Dr. Beverley Allan, *Australian Nurses Journal*, May 1978.

[39] Hannah Allen, *Don't Get Stuck: The Case Against Vaccinations...*, (Oldsmar, FL: Natural Hygiene Press, 1985), p. 144.

[40] PDR, pp. 1697-1699.

[41] Ibid and Attenuation of "RA 27/3 Rubella Virus in WI-38 Human Diploid Cells," *Amer. J. Dis. Child*, vol. 118, Aug. 1969, and "Studies of Immunization With Living Rubella Virus," *Arch. J. Dis. Child*, vol. 110, Oct. 1965.

[42] John Hanchette, "Safety of Controversial Hepatitis B Vaccine at Center of Debate," Gannett News Service, 5 May 1999.

[43] PDR, pp. 1744-1747 and 2482-2484.

[44] Ibid.

[45] PDR, pp. 1762-1765.

[46] Ibid.

[47] CDC Viral Hepatitis A, Fact Sheet, 29 Sept. 2000 (www.cdc.gov/ncidod/diseases/hepatitis/a/fact.htm).

[48] CDC Hepatitis A Vaccine, Vaccine Information Statement, 25 Aug. 1998.

[49] CDC Hepatitis A Facts, 16 Nov. 2000.

[50] Mosby's GenRX®, 10th ed., Hepatitis A Vaccine (003158) as posted on MDConsult website.

[51] CDC Hepatitis A Vaccine, Vaccine Information Statement, 25 Aug. 1998.

[52] Mosby's GenRX@, Hepatitis A Vaccine.

[53] Ibid.

[54] "Combined Hepatitis A/B Vaccine Offers Fast Protection," Reuters Health, 12 April 2000.

[55] Vaccines and Their Ingredients, 24 June 1999 (www.909shot.com).

[56] Michael Horwin, MA, "Prevnar: A Critical Review of a New Childhood Vaccine," 19 Sept. 2000.

[57] Prevnar package insert, Wyeth Lederle, 17 Feb. 2000.

[58] Ibid.

[59] Horwin, "Prevnar: A Critical Review."

[60] Dr. Erdem Cantekin, Ph.D., "Pneumococcal Vaccine and Otitis Media," NVIC's 2nd Intl. Public Conference, 8 Sept. 2000.

[61] Horwin, "Prevnar: A Critical Review."

[62] U. Parashar, C. Gibson, J. Bresee, and R. Glass, "Rotavirus and Severe Childhood Diarrhea," *Emerging Infectious Diseases*, 2006, 12(2). Available online: http://www,cdc.gov/ncidod/vol12no02/05-0006.htm

[63] U. Parashar, C. Gibson, J. Bresee, and R. Glass, "Hospitalizations Associated With Rotavirus Diarrhea in the United States, 1993 Through 1995: Surveillance Based on the New ICD-9CM Rotavirus-Specific Diagnostic Code," *Journal of Infectious Diseases*, 1198:177(1). Available online: http://www.journals. uchicago.edu/JID/Journal/issues/v177n1/ja07_13.web.pdf

[64] Null, Gary, "Vaccination: An Analysis of the Health Risks," Part 3, *Townsend Letter for Doctors and Patients*, Dec. 2003, p. 78.

[65] Research information available online: http://www.fda.gov/cber/safety/ phnrota021307.htm

[66] http://www.cdc.gov/index.htm

[67] http://www.fda.gov/cber/vaers/vaers.htm

[68] R. S. Paffenbarger, Jr., *JAMA* 27 Jul. 1984, 252(4):491-495.

[69] M. Messina, V. Messina, and K.D. Setchell, *The Simple Soybean and Your Health* (Garden City Park, NY: Avery Publishing Group, 1994) p. 24.

[70] H.M. Linkswiler, M.B. Zemel, et al., *Fed Proc*, Jul. 1981, 40(9):2429-2433.

[71] N.B. Belloc and L. Breslow, *Prev. Med*, Aug. 1972, 1(3):409-421.

[72] J.P. Carter and J. Brown, *Journal of the Louisiana State Medical Society*, 1985, 137(6):35-38.

[73] Richard A. Passwater, Ph.D., *Beta-Carotene: The Backstage Nutrient Now Universally Recognized for Cancer Prevention* (New Canaan, CT: Keats Publishing Inc., 1984).

[74] *The Lancet*, 1998, 3S 1.

[75] *American Journal of Ophthalmology*, 1997, p. 124.

[76] *The Lancet*, 1994, 343: 105.

[77] S.A. Beck, et al., "Egg Hypersensitivity and Measles-Mumps-Rubella Vaccine Administration," *Pediatrics*, Nov. 1991, 88(5):913-7.

[78] *The Lancet*, 1995, 346:1339-45.

[79] *Medical Monitor*, 5 June 1992.

[80] V. Romanus, R. Jonsell, and S.O. Bergquist, "Pertussis in Sweden After the Cessation of General Immunization in 1979," *Pediatr. Infect. Dis. J.*, 1987, 6(6):364.

Suggested Reading

DIET AND NUTRITION
Brackett, N., and Brackett, J., *Seven Secrets Cookbook* (Hagerstown, MD: Review and Herald Publishing Association, 2006).

Diehl, H., and Ludington, A., *An Ounce of Prevention* (Hagerstown, MD: Review and Herald Publishing Association, 2006).

Lawson, G., and Puffer, D., *Tasty Vegan Delights* (Hagerstown, MD: Review and Herald Publishing Association, 2001).

Scharffenberg, J. A., *Dietary Fat and Cholesterol* (Bakersfield, CA: Pacific Health Education Center, 1996).

Messina, M., and Messina, V., *The Dietitian's Guide to Vegetarian Diets* (Gaithersburg, MD: Aspen Publishers, Inc., 1996).

GENERAL REFERENCES
Austin, P., Thrash, A., and Thrash, C., *Natural Remedies: A Manual* (Sunfield, MI: Family Health Publications, LLC, 1983).

Austin, P., Thrash, A., and Thrash, C., *More Natural Remedies,* (Sunfield, MI: Family Health Publications, LLC, 1985).

McNeilus, M.A., *God's Healing Way* (Whalan, MN: Mercy Valley Farm, 2004).

White, E.G., *Counsels on Diet and Foods* (Hagerstown, MD: Review and Herald Publishing Association, multiple editions).

White, E.G., *The Use of Drugs in the Care of the Sick* (Middleton, ID: CHJ Publishing, 1954).

HERBAL MEDICINE
Hoffman, D., *Medical Herbalism, The Science and Practice of Herbal Medicine* (Rochester, VT: Healing Arts Press, 2003).

Duke, J.A., *The Green Pharmacy* (New York, NY: St. Martin's Press, 1998).

HYDROTHERAPY
Dail, C. and Thomas, C., *Hydrotherapy* (Brushton, NY: TEACH Service Inc., 1995).

MASSAGE
Kellogg, J. H., *The Art of Massage* (Brushton, NY: TEACH Service Inc., 1998).